W0113769

"Sex, faith, culture, and religion are often inextricably linked. Not always in seen or obvious ways but in no doubt within the therapeutic domain. In much of our work the blend of these aspects of the client's life needs to be included; to exclude them does the client a disservice. Dr. Caleb Jacobson's book gives the ability to speak in a meaningful and open way. It is an excellent resource for therapists to look through a religious lens in service to their clients."

Judi Keshet-Orr, MSc., *Founder and Course Director of The London Diploma in Psychosexual and Relationship Therapy*

"Dr. Caleb Jacobson's new book, *Sex Therapy with Religious Patients*, is a practical resource that will help sex therapists and students in training cultivate the cultural competencies necessary for ethical practice when working with conventionally religious clients. I look forward to having my students engage with this valuable text."

Mark A. Yarhouse, Psy.D., *Dr. Arthur P. Rech & Mrs. Jean May Rech Professor of Psychology and Director of the Sexual & Gender Identity Institute at Wheaton College*

"The intersection of religion and sex is often labeled as problematic or is left unaddressed in the therapeutic setting. Yet for religious clients, sexuality cannot be separated from their worldview. Dr. Caleb Jacobson's book is a powerful voice for these clients, and an indispensable resource for the therapists who serve them. Finally—sex is being spoken about from and through religious contexts in an empowering, bold, and practical manner."

Sameera Qureshi, M.S., *Sexual Health for Muslims*

Sex Therapy with Religious Patients

Sex Therapy with Religious Patients is a comprehensive guidebook for mental health professionals who work with those struggling with sexual issues within a religious context. The book provides practical guidance on how to approach sensitive topics related to sex and religion, including addressing religious beliefs and values that may impact sexual behavior, beliefs, and attitudes.

Drawing on research and clinical experience, the book offers a range of evidence-based interventions for working with individuals from different Jewish, Christian, and Muslim backgrounds. It also explores the unique challenges and opportunities presented by patients' religious beliefs and provides strategies for integrating spirituality into the therapeutic process.

The book is written in an accessible and engaging style, with real-life case examples and exercises that can be used in therapy sessions. It is an essential resource for mental health professionals seeking to enhance their skills in working with religious individuals who are seeking sex therapy.

Caleb Jacobson, PsyD, PhD, is an internationally recognized clinical psychologist, sex therapist, and Bible scholar. Currently, he serves as president of both the School of Sex Therapy and the International Association of Psychosexual Therapists.

Sex Therapy with Religious Patients

Working with Jewish, Christian, and Muslim Communities

Caleb Jacobson

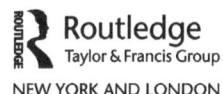

Routledge
Taylor & Francis Group

NEW YORK AND LONDON

Designed cover: aelitta © Getty Images

First published 2024
by Routledge
605 Third Avenue, New York, NY 10158

and by Routledge
4 Park Square, Milton Park, Abingdon, Oxon, OX14 4RN

Routledge is an imprint of the Taylor & Francis Group, an informa business

© 2024 Caleb Jacobson

The right of Caleb Jacobson to be identified as author of this work has been asserted in accordance with sections 77 and 78 of the Copyright, Designs and Patents Act 1988.

All rights reserved. No part of this book may be reprinted or reproduced or utilised in any form or by any electronic, mechanical, or other means, now known or hereafter invented, including photocopying and recording, or in any information storage or retrieval system, without permission in writing from the publishers.

Trademark notice: Product or corporate names may be trademarks or registered trademarks, and are used only for identification and explanation without intent to infringe.

Library of Congress Cataloging-in-Publication Data
Names: Jacobson, Caleb, author.
Title: Sex therapy with religious patients : working with Jewish, Christian, and Muslim communities / Caleb Jacobson.
Description: New York, NY : Routledge, 2024. | Includes bibliographical references and index.
Identifiers: LCCN 2023054826 (print) | LCCN 2023054827 (ebook) | ISBN 9781032149738 (hbk) | ISBN 9781032149721 (pbk) | ISBN 9781003242017 (ebk)
Subjects: LCSH: Sex therapy—Religious aspects. | Sex—Religious aspects.
Classification: LCC RC557 .J33 2024 (print) | LCC RC557 (ebook) | DDC 616.85/8306—dc23/eng/20240209
LC record available at https://lccn.loc.gov/2023054826
LC ebook record available at https://lccn.loc.gov/2023054827

ISBN: 978-1-032-14973-8 (hbk)
ISBN: 978-1-032-14972-1 (pbk)
ISBN: 978-1-003-24201-7 (ebk)

DOI: 10.4324/9781003242017

Typeset in Palatino
by Apex CoVantage, LLC

Support Material is available for this title at www.routledge.com/9781032149738

Dedication

לאהבה
תודה שתמכת בי בכל מה שאני עושה.

Contents

Acknowledgements

The creation of this book has been a collaborative effort, and there are many individuals I'd like to express my gratitude to.

First and foremost, I want to extend my heartfelt thanks to my family. I realize that explaining to others that your child or sibling is both a Bible scholar and a sex therapist can be complex, and my unpredictable public statements may raise eyebrows at times. Your unwavering support, even when you may not fully comprehend my endeavors, has been an incredible source of empowerment. I love each one of you dearly.

I would like to acknowledge Dr. Richelle Dadian for her dedication to this project, often putting in extra hours, even when rest would have been more welcoming, to contribute to the book's production. Thank you. I truly value your friendship.

To Sameera Qureshi, your friendship has been a true inspiration. Your consistent support for my work means the world to me, and I am deeply grateful to have you in my corner.

My sincere appreciation goes out to Rivka Sidorsky for her willingness to review and provide feedback on sections of the book. Your insights have been valuable, and I treasure your friendship and support.

Together, your contributions and encouragement have played a significant role in bringing this book to fruition.

Introduction

Introduction

Sex and religion are often seen as mutually exclusive and combining the two seem paradoxical. This can frequently be observed in the therapeutic process when the religious views of the patient, or even that of the therapist, appear to introduce concepts or attitudes that are contrary to that which is conducive to ethical and efficacious therapy. Likewise, perhaps no other environmental and cultural influence is more readily met with bias on the part of the therapist than that of religion, wherein a patient's religious beliefs are sometimes understood as the cause of the presenting problem resulting in emotional distress and sometimes labeled as harmful. Such tension leads to feelings of frustration experienced by both the therapist and the patient.

It is not unusual for a therapist to feel anxious in navigating sexual issues with religious patients, nor is it uncommon for religious patients to feel trepidation in even discussing such topics. Yet, areas of sex, sexuality, and gender are just as influential and impactful facets of the human experience in the lives of religious patients as they are to their nonreligious counterparts. The major difference is that the religious views of the patient may be contrary to the cultural norms and societal views of any given time. Additionally, religious patients normally receive little to no sex education, making the requirement for psychosexual education even more necessary.

DOI: 10.4324/9781003242017-1

Despite the conflict between the two subjects, or perhaps, *because* of the conflict between the two, the topics of sex and religion are rather popular. This phenomenon is not new. In fact, it has been a continual theme in pop culture. Think of Elvis, whose onstage moves were considered sexually provocative at the time, and yet he would always incorporate gospel songs into his performance. Or consider the connotations of the song titled "Like A Virgin" being sung by an artist named Madonna. The fascination of combining the two is perhaps linked to the perceived, and sometimes real, conflict that exists within the subjects thus being viewed as taboo.

The fascination between sex and religion is not limited to pop culture. It frequently invades the sphere of academics in psychology, biblical studies, and sex and gender studies. Consider the number of titles written on the psychology of religion. Or, consider that the leading professional organization for biblical scholars, the Society of Biblical Literature, offers several sessions on the topic of "Gender, Sexuality, and the Bible" at their annual conference. Such publications and areas of academic research should be of little surprise considering the massive motivational factor that both sexuality and religion have played throughout history.

Acknowledging the significant ascendancy that both sex and religion hold, it can be expected that clinicians will encounter patients confronted with opposing ideologies. While many, if not most, sex therapists can recall instances when a patient's religious worldview was the cause of their emotional distress, it is cautioned that religion should not be viewed as the antagonist. In fact, within these pages, it is argued that addressing the beliefs of the patient in such a manner is overall counterproductive and can be dangerous to the patient's well-being. Instead, it is suggested that the religious worldview of the patient be taken into consideration and used within the therapeutic process whenever possible in order to employ a more holistic approach to treatment, relying on systems that have already been developed and established within the patient's life. Yet, working within such a framework can be perceived as a difficult, if not impossible, task for the therapist.

This volume aims to provide valuable resources to clinicians working with religious patients by providing relevant details on the religious practices of Jewish, Christian, and Muslim believers and demonstrating how to work with these individuals and couples through common issues in sex therapy in an ethical manner that respects their religious worldview. Unlike some of the texts and trainings that have previously been available, the goal of this book is to avoid generalizations and distinguish between the orthodox and liberal adherers within each of these Abrahamic faiths and recognize the unique perspectives they bring.

In order to make the most out of this text, it has been divided into four sections to act as a frequent resource. Part I provides a theoretical understanding of the role religion has on the development and worldview of the patient and highlights some of the often overlooked issues that religious patients have about participating in sex therapy. Within this section, you will also discover ways to help the patient feel more at ease during the initial contact and ways to make the first session relaxed and comfortable. Protocol for working with religious patients will also be provided.

Part II of this book aims to offer essential insights into the religious beliefs and perspectives on diverse sexual topics held by Jews, Christians, and Muslims. Serving as a valuable reference, it provides key terms specific to each faith tradition, enabling practitioners to understand their patients and communicate in a manner that fosters relaxation and avoids feelings of threat or discomfort. The three chapters delve into the broad belief systems within each faith, emphasizing the importance of acknowledging the wide range of individual beliefs within each religious community to prevent generalizations based solely on religious affiliation. By exploring these distinct religious perspectives, practitioners can better understand their patients' religious context and engage in culturally sensitive and respectful conversations about sexuality.

Common issues within sex therapy are presented in Part III of this book. For each of the topics, actual cases are provided as examples, though names and specific identifying details have been omitted or changed. These chapters also provide reference to sacred texts, which are commonly used to establish belief systems concerning the topic discussed, and texts for further reading are provided to be used as tools within the therapeutic process. Each of these chapters demonstrates the necessity of using the PLISSIT (Permission, Limited Information, Specific Suggestions, Intense Therapy) model and demonstrates how to integrate it within each context.

Part IV of this book addresses concerns that therapists may have when working with patients who have belief systems that are antithetical to their own. It emphasizes the importance of ethics in the mental and behavioral health field and how therapist bias can be dangerous to the patient. It also points out the bias of the patient, which can present within the therapeutic alliance. Tips on overcoming bias are given; as well as encouragement when dealing with the very real, very difficult, and sometimes very frustrating situations that arise when practicing sex therapy with religious individuals and couples.

Finally, three very useful appendixes are provided at the conclusion of this book. The glossary of terms contains not only the key terms highlighted in Chapters 3–5, but also additional terms that are part of the common vernacular of each religion discussed. This will help foster greater understanding and communication with the patient. The second appendix consists of reflection questions to help therapists recognize areas of bias that they may have. The final appendix is a list of resources that may prove to be helpful when further exploring sex and religion, both in the therapeutic setting and for means of professional development. These resources can be used by the therapist and patient alike.

As you delve into this book, please consider the following. Within therapeutic circles, we often talk about the necessity of working with marginalized groups. Nowhere is this rhetoric heard more than among sex therapists. Yet, it is not uncommon to hear disenfranchising commitments made about religious groups or belief systems spoken by members of these same crowds. But should we not view religious patients who come to sex therapy as marginalized? The topic is mostly foreign to religious patients. Resources and support typically required throughout the therapeutic process are unattainable. And lest we forget, many times these patients come to us often as outcasts, often abused (physically, mentally, emotionally, sexually, spiritually), sometimes traumatized, many times rejected, and often fearful of losing their entire social network of friends and family. Thus, I have no hesitation in labeling religious patients, in terms of sex therapy, as a marginalized population. It is a population that we must tirelessly work with and advocate for, just as we would any other marginalized group.

Having worked with a diverse group of religious patients in multiple countries with various languages, I have become all too familiar with the challenges that commonly arise in sex therapy when working with religious individuals and couples. However, I also know the rewards of such efforts. My journey is quite unique in that I work both as a sex therapist and as a Hebrew Bible scholar. This has allowed me unique opportunities to explore topics, texts, and other resources often unavailable or impractical for others to study. It has also made me aware of the desire for a comprehensive resource on tackling tough topics of sex, sexuality, and gender within religious communities.

It is with great hope that clinicians, who have previously struggled in their work with religious patients, will feel better equipped in future encounters and, in the process, offer a more comfortable and understanding environment in which religious patients are able to flourish in the therapeutic work. While working with such a population may present its own distinctive challenges, the process is an exceptionally rewarding one in which you can observe both the growth of the patient and your professional growth as a sex therapist. It is with this aspiration that *Sex Therapy with Religious Patients* was written.

Dr. Caleb Jacobson, PsyD, PhD
Mainz, Germany
October 2023

PART I

Sex, Religion, and the Therapeutic Process

Overview

Within this section, readers will gain insight into the profound influence of religion on patient development and the intricate dynamics that may challenge the therapeutic alliance between clinician and patient. Moreover, readers will be equipped with a meticulously structured protocol for effectively engaging with religious patients, alongside invaluable recommendations to enhance the overall therapeutic experience.

Learning Objectives

+ Name three ways that a therapist's bias projects toward religious patients.
+ Identify at least three areas where religion and culture intersect.
+ Recall at least two fears religious patients have when seeking sex therapy.
+ Explain the four steps in the Jacobson Model.

DOI: 10.4324/9781003242017-2

1

Working with Religious Patients

Introduction

Truth be told, most therapists feel unprepared to work with religious patients. The topics of sex, sexuality, and gender are already quite diverse, and issues related to these topics are complicated and complex. Then you must consider religion. Religion on its own is also extremely diverse, with various denominations and sects within each faith group, all of which have differing dogmas and theological beliefs that can make them radically different from other groups who also profess the same religious faith. When you combine the two, it can become a rather difficult terrain to navigate. Yet, this is the path that the therapist, who most likely has no theological training or knowledge, must try and guide their patient through.

This is not an easy task, even for the most astute therapist. Despite the way it is often perceived, religion is not monolithic, even among particular faith groups (Friedman, 2019). Many clinicians would automatically recognize that there are differing belief systems among Jews, Christians, and Muslims, but what about the diversity within each of these groups? Christianity, as an example, has the most subsects of any faith tradition. There is a big difference in the beliefs and practices between fundamentalist Christians, such as the Southern Baptists, and more liberal-leaning sects, such as the United Church of Christ. To make matters even more complicated, there is great diversity

DOI: 10.4324/9781003242017-3

even within fundamentalist sects and among churches with the same denominational title. For example, within Apostolic Pentecostalism, some churches may forbid young couples to hold hands, kiss, or even sit next to each other; while others within the same denomination will make such allowances. All of this adds to the complexity of discussing sexual or gender-related issues with religious patients and can leave the clinician feeling ill-prepared.

In each of these cases, the patient's worldview introduces hurdles that must be skillfully maneuvered. The term "worldview" is often uncomfortable and unsettling for many sex therapists. This is because most sex therapists would have difficulty using the term in correlation with sexual orientation. They would argue that a person's sexual orientation is not a worldview. However, a religious patient who is conservative or fundamentalist would most likely disagree and would, in fact, consider it a worldview. The sex therapist must then make a choice, risk losing the patient by trying to persuade them to the therapist's point of view or adopt the language that the patient uses. It should be noted that the term "worldview" is widely used in the greater field of clinical psychology (Mudryk & Johnson, 2022). The term is also used within the specific modality of cognitive behavioral therapy (Naeem et al., 2023). Therefore, it is recommended that without hesitation, the clinician adopt the patient vernacular (Chandler et al., 2019).

Herein lies another obstacle that commonly arises when working with religious patients – the therapist's bias. This occurs most often when the worldview of the clinician is counter to the worldview of the patient. There are numerous reasons why this could happen. For example, the clinician could simply feel that the beliefs held by the patient are problematic. Frequently, therapists have commented to me that their patient's belief "just isn't good for them." And in a climate where social justice and activism have radically infiltrated therapeutic practice, some therapists have no problems confronting patients about their religious belief system. However, this is an extremely dangerous practice and one that will cause religious patients to abandon treatment as it solidifies the bias the patient already has about therapy, as will be seen in the next chapter.

Another recurrent phenomenon related to therapist bias is connected to the clinician's own religious background. It is not uncommon to discover that a sex therapist has entered the specialty due to negative and often traumatic religious experiences that they themselves encountered. This can range from sexual guilt and shame imposed by stringent Purity Culture teachings, to isolation, abandonment, and rejection due to their sexual orientation. While it is understandable that these experiences have given the clinician a negative view of religion, this bias

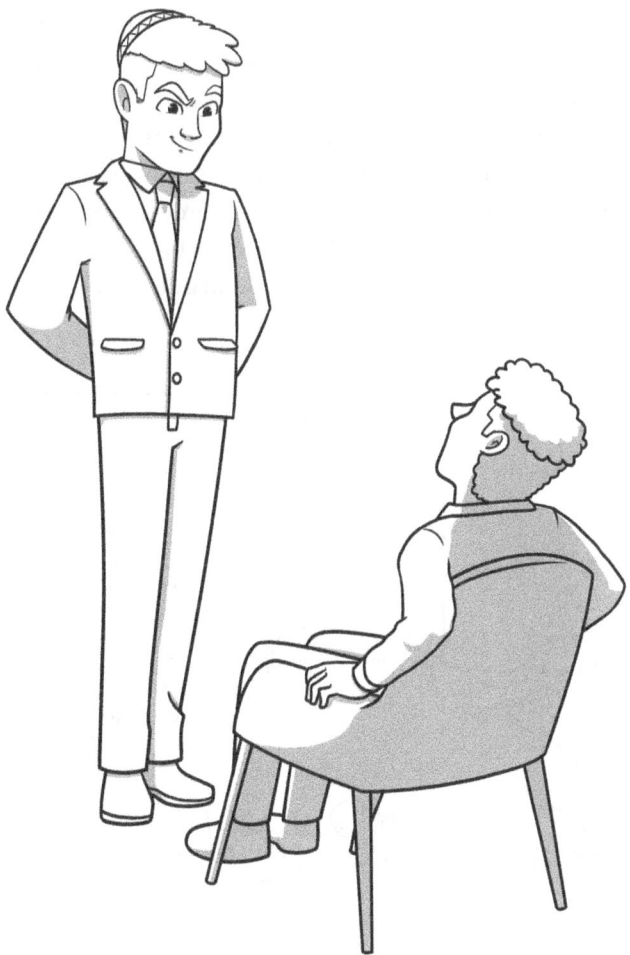

FIGURE 1.1 The therapist above the patient.

manifests itself far too often within the therapeutic relationship. In speaking with patients, therapist bias usually presents itself in one of three ways: (1) The therapist above the patient, (2) the therapist as the patient, and (3) the therapist against the patient.

The therapist above the patient refers to a sense of superiority that the therapist feels over their religious patient. Cognitively, they believe they have reached a higher level of enlightenment than their patient. The clinician may even pity the religious patient for holding on to such "primitive beliefs" (an expression relayed by a patient). This bias manifests itself within the therapeutic setting, most often as condescension.

The therapist as the patient refers to a clinician projecting their experience onto the patient. In this situation, the therapist sees common variables within the patient's narrative and their own personal experience and feels the need to interfere. Commonly, this is motivated by the conscious or unconscious wish of the clinician that someone would have interfered in their past experience. This bias manifests itself whereby the clinician feels they must rescue their patient from their destructive religious beliefs.

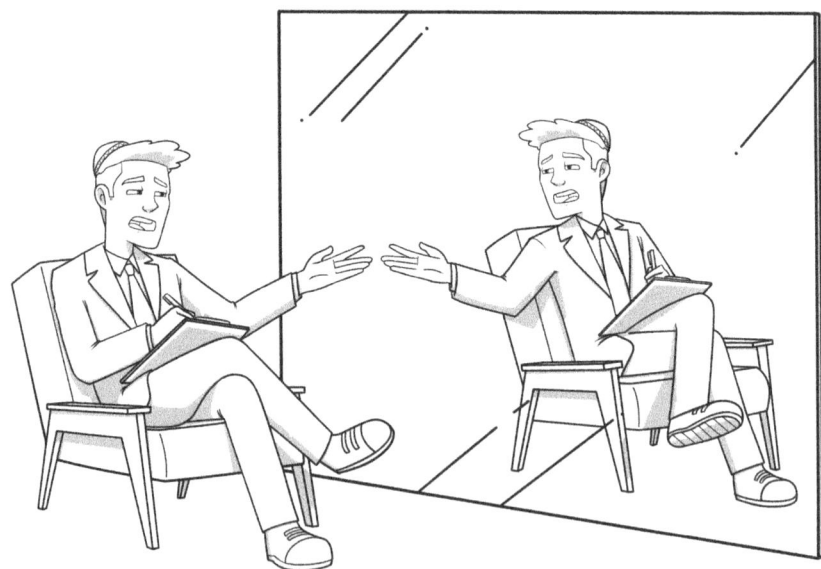

FIGURE 1.2 The therapist as the patient.

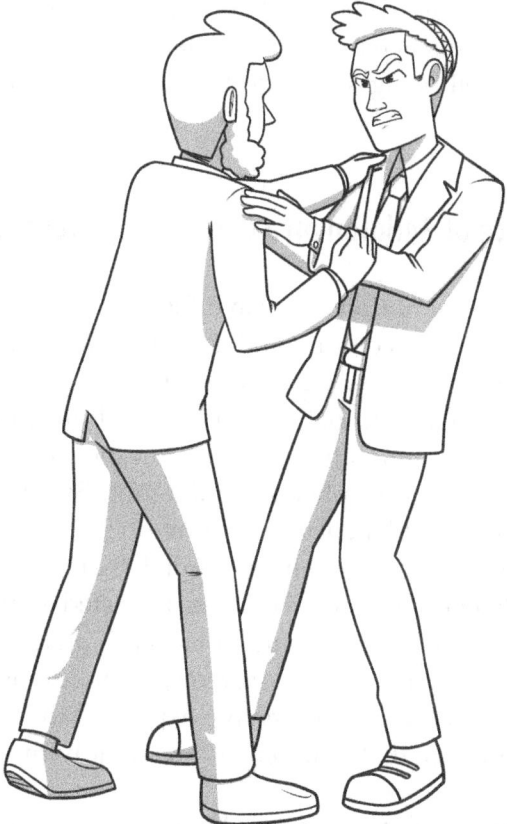

FIGURE 1.3 The therapist against the patient.

The therapist against the patient refers to the clinician viewing the patient as the embodiment of their previous trauma. In other words, the religious patient is the symbol of every negative thing that has previously happened to the therapist. This bias usually manifests itself as hostility and resentment toward the patient.

While all three of these biases appear different, the crux of each is the belief that religion is bad and that it negatively impacts the patient, and as such, it is the source of their core problem(s). And in a move that defies ethics, therapists, in these scenarios, will often tell their patients that their religion is the problem. Some even go as far as to tell the patient that they must leave their religious community and abandon their set of beliefs altogether if they ever hope to overcome their presenting issues. However, in most cases, this is extremely problematic and counter to the welfare and well-being of the individual or couple that they are working with.

The Influence of Religion on a Person's Development

Suggesting that an individual leave their religious faith ignores how deeply religious culture and community impact and influence their development. Developing greater insight into these spheres of influence is helpful to realize how problematic it can be to suggest to a patient to abandon their faith. In gaining such insight into these spheres of influence, **Bronfrenbrenner's Ecological Systems Theory** may prove helpful. Kitchen et al. (2019) explain, "Bronfenbrenner argued that humans actively engage with evolving, interconnected, nested environments." While this text does not permit an in-depth analysis of each of these nested environments or systems, some important aspects should be briefly touched on before exploring the multi-faceted sphere of influence that religion has on an individual.

A Brief History of Ecological Systems Theory

Bronfenbrenner developed his theory as a way to understand the numerous variables that impact the development of a person over time. As Smart (2019, 495) stated, "Freud characterized humans as closed systems; Erikson included society's expectations as one source of motivation; but it was Bronfenbrenner who characterized humans as open systems that interact with the environment." Therefore, the core of systems theory is the individual with their own unique set of characteristics and qualities, such as their biological sex, their health, and other genetic and biological dispositions. These are all unique and individual to the specific person at the system's center.

The system closest to the individual is the **microsystem**. The microsystem is made up of the interactions and relationships that have the most direct influence on the person. For example, a person's family, their partner or spouse, and close friends all fall

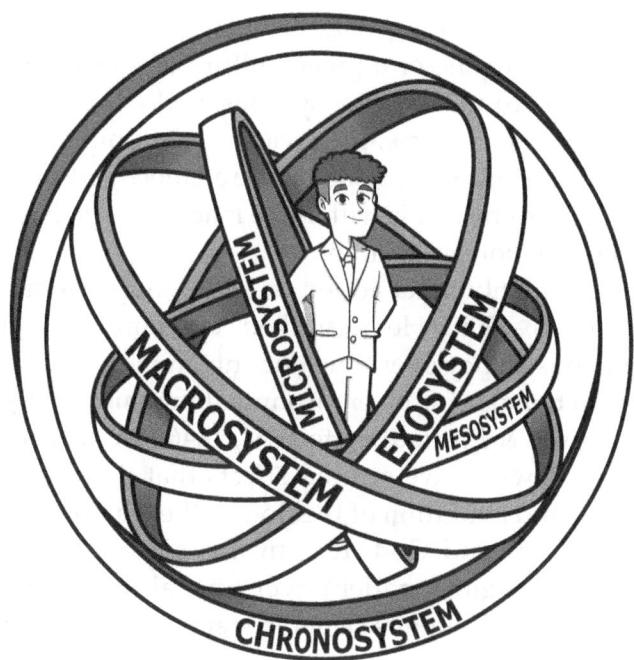

FIGURE 1.4 Ecological Systems Theory.

within the microsystem. Additionally, Bronfenbrenner stated that besides the face-to-face encounters, the interaction a person has with the world of symbols and language are also included in the microsystem (Bronfenbrenner, 2005, xvii). For a religious patient, this could mean the sacred text, images related to their faith tradition, and the language used by their specific faith community.

Following the microsystem is the **exosystem**. This system includes one or more systems that do not have direct involvement with the individual. Bronfenbrenner (2005, xiii) used the example of a parent's workplace and the effect that it indirectly has on a developing child since it interferes with their parent's availability and impact on their parent's stress level (Bronfenbrenner, 2005, xiii). For the religious person, this system would also include their house of worship (synagogue, church, mosque) as well as religious community centers.

Next is the **macrosystem**. Colwell, Pollard, and Pollard (2015, 161) described it best when they stated, "The macrosystem consists of the overarching pattern of micro-, meso-, and the ecosystem characteristic of a given culture or subculture, with particular reference to the belief systems, bodies of knowledge, material resources, customs, life-styles, opportunity structures, hazards, and life course options that are embedded in each of those broader systems." It is within the macrosystem that we see the impact of religion and culture.

Finally, Bronfenbrenner added an additional system known as the **chronosystem**. He described the chronosystem as, "change or consistency over time not only in the characteristics of the person but also of the environment in which that person lives …" (Husen & Postlethwaite 1994, 1646). In the context of religion, this is where we see the effects that time has on the development and evolution of theology – the way people think about and understand God. It is in this system that we see changes in the religious patient over time also, as they move in relation to their religious belief systems over the course of their life.

As ecological systems theory demonstrates, religion has a great impact on a person's development as it is present in every system that they encounter. For a religious person, every sphere of influence somehow touches their faith tradition. Religion does not just impact an individual's beliefs concerning sex, but also the way that they approach and understand the world in which they live. This is why many religious scholars and theologians use the term **worldview** to describe the lens through which a religious person understands the way that their beliefs differ from the general culture and society (Cook, 2021).

Two Aspects of Religious Influence: Text and Community

When conceptualizing the impact of religion on the individual, two aspects of religious influence should be considered. The first is the sacred text(s) of the particular religion. These texts are often considered to be divinely **inspired**, meaning that they were given by God directly or through a human vessel. The more fundamental the patient is, the more likely they are to believe that their sacred text is also **infallible**, meaning that the text does not include any errors.

Those who hold to the infallibility of their sacred texts would argue that any discrepancies found within are a result of copy errors or translation of the text and not transmission. In other words, a Christian patient may argue that perceived discrepancies in the New Testament are a result of translation from Greek to English (or some other language). They would argue that when the text was originally given and transcribed by the human author, it was done so without any error that could be visible in the text today.

The second aspect to consider is the unique religious community in which the person is a member. It is often necessary to distinguish between what a sacred text may say and the way in which a particular religious community interprets and applies that text. It is not uncommon, even within a particular denomination or sect, for communities to emphasize different texts and to have different standards of application. For example, a community may have consequences for engaging in sexual behavior outside of marriage; however, what those consequences are and how sexual behavior outside of marriage is defined is dependent on that particular community. This speaks to the autonomy of the individual communities. It is but one reason to inquire about the patient's understanding of certain fundamental issues as they relate to sex, sexuality, and gender, and not simply to assume based upon the clinician's previous experience working with religious individuals.

The role of the community in determining the application of texts for their members also carries psychological ramifications. As we have seen from Bronfenbrenner's ecological systems theory, a religious community does impact the development of an individual. The clergy has a major role in both the atmosphere, development, and direction of the community as a whole, as well as the sense of belonging and acceptance of the individual member. When it comes to the authority of the clergy, many fundamentalist and conservative religious groups, regardless of faith tradition, believe such authority comes from God. Sacred texts are often used to back such claims as well. While there may be some credence to the argument, this scenario is potentially hazardous and can lead to a spiritual dictatorship. In such cases, but certainly not all, spiritual abuse is prevalent.

In the context of sexual health and wellness, it is not uncommon for people to connect their religious experience to the guilt and shame that they have about sex. As a clinician, it is important to delineate between a particular religion and a particular religious community. In other words, a community may hold beliefs that are not found within their sacred texts. For example, Catholics believe in the concept of **purgatory**, though it is not something found within the biblical texts. Therefore, when working with religious patients, we must understand if the source of their issues is related to what their sacred texts say or a particular teaching of their faith tradition or community that is not necessarily based on sacred texts.

Religion and Culture

When examining the impact of religion on individuals and societies, it is crucial to acknowledge the interplay between religion and culture. Religion and culture are not mutually exclusive entities but rather closely intertwined, with significant overlap between them. Even in cases where religion and culture may not directly coincide, actions within one sphere often reflect responses from the other. Thus, it is essential to consider additional variables within the realm of religious influence, recognizing the intricate relationship between religion and culture and how they mutually shape beliefs, practices, and behaviors. By understanding this dynamic interplay, we gain a more comprehensive understanding of the complexities and nuances involved in the intersection of religion and culture.

Let us first consider that religion, and in particular individual religious communities, often have their own culture. As therapists, it is crucial to differentiate between the beliefs, actions, and theology of a particular religious community and its teachings, compared to the actual teachings and sacred texts of a particular religion. These can be two very distinct and separate

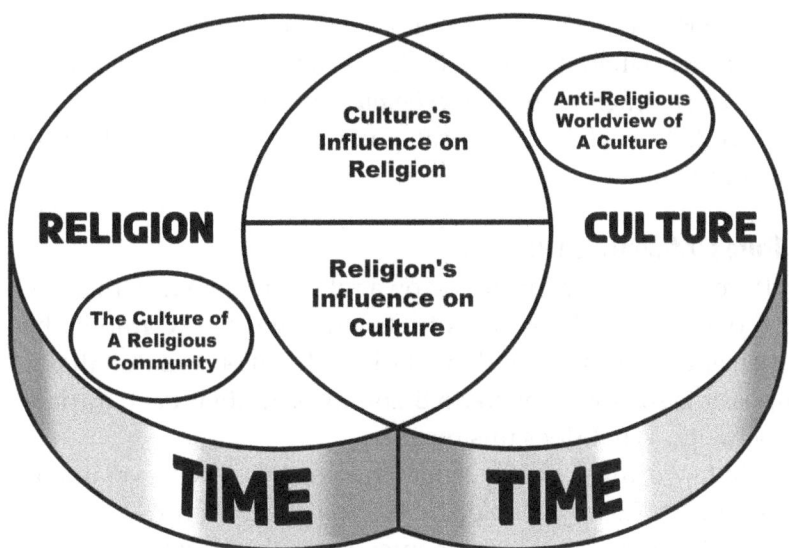

FIGURE 1.5 Intersection of religion and culture.

things. This is why it is often necessary to distinguish between the teachings of a particular community and the impact that it has on the individual and the teachings of the actual faith that they profess to practice.

Culture, on the other hand, can often have anti-religious views (at least in the mind of the religious patient). For example, we must consider restrictions that certain countries have on religious freedoms or the outright prohibition against religion or particular religious groups. This is yet one reason why sex therapists should view religious patients as part of a marginalized and disenfranchised group. Furthermore, for the religious patient, any political advancement, law, or action that appears to be an attack on any of their religious convictions is interpreted as an attack on their faith. Herein is another reason why therapists need to be mindful of self-disclosure. While you may be compelled to let your voice be heard when a patient has strong convictions against things such as abortion or gay rights, your activism and advocacy will only fall on deaf ears and cause hostility between you and the patient.

Nevertheless, there is a unique correlation between religion and culture, where the two overlap. Within this area, the *culture's influence on religion* and the *religion's influence on culture* can be observed. In each of these categories, the path of influence is multidirectional.

Culture's Influence on Religion

Culture plays a great influence on a religion in the way that a religion develops and responds to its surroundings. Catholic theologian and priest Johann Baptist Metz (1990) once stated that it is impossible for someone to do theology with their back turned to Auschwitz. What does this mean?

First, we must clarify what theology is. As I explained in *Handbook of Reading Theological German* (Jacobson & Hirt, 2021, 3–4), "The term "theology" comes from the Greek words Θεός (Theos, "God"), and λόγος (logos, "word," "speech," or "expression"). Thus, the term "theology" means a word about God. Or, to put it in more common terms, it is a conversation about God. Therefore, when anyone dialogues about their perspective or conception of God, they are in fact doing theology, regardless of their educational or religious background (even if they have neither)."

From this, we can understand that Metz was simply pointing out that the way that we think about God is influenced by our environment and history. In the context in which he was speaking, the Shoah challenged many people's theological beliefs concerning God. For example, if God is good, how could he allow something so bad to happen? This is something that many theologians wrestled with in the twentieth century.

Culture also challenges the way in which a religion is practiced. Historically, if we look at Jews in the diaspora, we can see how religious practices and languages were developed based on the location in which they lived – most notably the evolution of Ashkenazi and Sephardic Jewry (Olszewska et al., 2019). Similarly, it can be observed the way Catholicism is practiced in various South American countries is different than in other predominantly Catholic countries such as Ireland and Italy. Likewise, a faith tradition such as Islam, which contains massive ethnic diversity, will contain differences in the way a person lives out their faith based upon their geographic location and the culture that informs it (Reitsma, 2020).

Religion's Influence on Culture

Religion also has an influence on culture. Many people of faith are informed by their religious convictions when they exercise their right to vote. This cannot be seen clearer than the election of Ronald Reagan in 1981 with the help of Baptist minister Rev. Jerry Falwell and his coalition known as the Moral Majority (Shupe & Stacey, 1982). Similarly, many credit Evangelical Christians for the election of Donald Trump (Miller, 2019; Holder & Josephson, 2020). Some scholars have gone so far as to suggest the theological implications arguing that Evangelicals were able to identify with Trump's negative worldviews by replacing postmillennialism with premillennial theology (Myers, 2019).

There is also an interesting correlation point of cross-influence between culture and religion. In the book *Abrahamic Faiths: Perspectives on Gender Identity and Sexuality* (Jacobson, 2023), I discuss how a cultural idea and concept, like Victorianism, was adopted by the church. While the concepts were largely rejected by British people, the ideology spread to other continents, cultures, and countries by Christian missionaries. Thus demonstrating a unique phenomenon of how religion spreads an idea that it adopted, not from its religious texts or historical theology, but from culture.

Religion evolves as a direct result of culture. As groups within a faith tradition respond to the world around them – adopting or opposing cultural norms and societal views, the religious community changes. This is one explanation for the numerous denominations and sects within a particular tradition. Additionally, as demonstrated, it also explains why there is such diversity even within those sects. While this may make working with religious individuals and couples seem more complicated, it actually provides a window of opportunity for being inquisitive and learning about their faith journey and their relationship to their faith tradition. It also allows clinicians to get a better grasp of the nuances and specifics that have led them to seek therapy.

Discerning the Problem: Ethical Considerations

Because religious beliefs and religious community have been important variables in the development and personhood of the patient, it is clear to see how instructing them to abandon their faith is not always in their best interest. Granted, there are instances where such advice is warranted, primarily when there is physical, sexual, or spiritual abuse that is taking place. But even in these instances, the advice is not for the patient to abandon their religion but to find a new religious community. It is far too easy for the practitioner to over-generalize and blame religion itself for all of the patient's issues (or even the issues that they have had in their past) instead of recognizing and identifying the specific trauma that took place. However, this is a bit unfair.

If a patient were in an abusive relationship, physical or sexual, the clinician would probably recommend that they get out of that relationship and leave their partner. It would not cross the mind of the therapist to suggest to their patient to never date again and stay away from all relationships. The reasoning is simple. The therapist recognizes that abuse is taking place in this particular relationship. They have named and identified the abuse. Relationships are not the patient's problem. The patient's problem is abuse. Yet, this same clarity is lacking when it comes to religion.

There is no doubt that abuse takes place within religious communities. The abuse can be physical, psychological, emotional, sexual, or spiritual, although the last rarely gets discussed. In these instances, it should be recognized that it is rarely the religion itself that is the abusive factor, but rather the abuse comes from an environment that has been created through selfishness and the manipulation of religious texts. This is similar to an abusive relationship. The construct of a relationship is not abusive in itself. However, with the addition of selfishness and the manipulation of emotions, it can be very abusive and problematic.

This distinction between religion and religious community must be made clear. Regardless of if the patient decides it is in their best interest to stay in their religious community or to leave, the ethical sex therapist will seek ways to support their patient in finding congruency between their spiritual beliefs and their sexual attitudes. It would be ethically irresponsible to automatically assert that an individual or couple should leave their community, as such a suggestion does not take into account the various influences already mentioned, as well as the environment and daily living structure they have created for themselves. Leaving their faith could mean losing their family, losing their friends, and losing their sense of self-identity.

In certain religious traditions, particularly Judaism and Islam, faith takes on a very collectivist role – more so than in Christianity.[1] Christianity, in terms of its religious tradition and sacred texts, is best described as an individualist culture. There are some New Testament texts that would support the idea of a communal faith. For example, Hebrews 10:24–25, "And let us consider how to stir up one another to love and good works, *not neglecting to meet together*, as is the habit of some, but encouraging one another and all the more as you see the Day drawing near" (English Standard Version Bible, 2018, italics added). The Apostle Paul, writer of roughly one-fourth of the New Testament, discussed the importance of the Church coming together as a collective to better one another (English Standard Version Bible, 2018, 1 Corinthians 11:17–22). However, Christianity, unlike Judaism, for example, is still much more individualistic due to its emphasis on individual salvation. Take, for example, Paul's encouragement that Christians should be less concerned with their own interest but of the interest of others (English Standard Version Bible, 2018, Philippians 2:4) yet continues by saying, "work out *your own salvation* with fear and trembling" (English Standard Version Bible, 2018, Philippians 2:12, italics inserted).

Nevertheless, all three Abrahamic faith traditions are considered ethno-religious groups. People who are a part of these faith traditions embody these systems as part of their identity. As Darshefsky (1972, 243) long ago reported, "Identification [is] viewed both as a process upon which identity is elaborated and as a product of social interactions." Therefore, when a therapist suggests that a patient abandon their faith tradition, they are also suggesting that they abandon their worldview, which is connected to their self-identity and social interactions. Thus, it becomes a dangerous prescription that can cause the patient to spiral into crisis mode, unsure of who they are, what they believe, or what direction their future is headed.

Bringing Religion into the Therapy Room

Besides the possible breach of ethics involved in telling a patient to leave their religious faith, such instruction is usually not necessary and causes more problems than it does solutions. In fact, it can be exceptionally useful to incorporate the patient's religious beliefs into the therapeutic process. Besides being an integral part of a holistic approach to treatment, religion can be, and often is, a helpful resource for clinicians – despite the perception. This is because religion offers three components that are exceptionally helpful in the therapeutic process: (1) A support system, (2) a positive outlook, (3) and a sense of purpose.

Support System

The mental and behavioral health profession has long recognized the value of support systems in aiding the patient to reach their goals (Harandi, Taghinasab, & Nayeri, 2017). Patients who come from a religious community have a pre-established support system within their religious community. This network can be leveraged within the clinical arena to aid in the patient's treatment. Kim, Sherman, and Taylor (2008), conducted a study that acknowledged the benefit of a support system in dealing with something such as stress but specifically highlighted the role of support systems within individual cultures. Therefore, a clinician can utilize the religio-ethnic culture of their faith tradition and individual community to provide support for individuals and couples who are navigating difficult emotional, psychological, and behavioral health challenges.

Positive Outlook

During times of crisis, individuals often find even the simplest tasks challenging to navigate. Their optimism wanes, along with their motivation, determination, and desire to overcome the hurdles they encounter, sometimes leading to a loss of hope in life itself. This negative thinking can have detrimental effects on a person's mental health (Fonseca & Canavarro, 2020). Conversely, maintaining a positive outlook can have a beneficial impact on mental well-being (Laranjeira & Querido, 2022).

Numerous studies have consistently shown a relationship between religion and optimism (Warren et al., 2015; Reynolds et al., 2019). In fact, research suggests that individuals with more fundamentalist religious beliefs tend to exhibit higher levels of optimism (Sethi & Seligman, 1993). This optimism can serve as a valuable asset within the therapeutic process, particularly in the context of sex therapy when working with couples who perceive their sexual issues as negatively affecting the future of their relationship. By incorporating and harnessing the power of optimism, clinicians can help these couples cultivate a hopeful outlook, fostering resilience and motivation to overcome their challenges. Recognizing the potential influence of religious beliefs and their associated optimism provides a valuable resource in guiding both individuals and couples toward healing and a brighter future within their sexual and relational lives.

Sense of Purpose

Religion also adds a sense of purpose to one's life. Religious patients often feel that they were created and placed on this earth for a specific purpose. This mentality is deeply rooted in the biblical text. Take, for example, the following passage of scripture: "For if you keep silent at this time, relief and deliverance will rise for the Jews from another place, but you and your father's house will perish. And who knows whether you have not come to the kingdom for such a time as this?" (English Standard Version Bible, 2018, Esther 4:14).

A patient's sense of purpose plays a crucial role in the therapeutic process, offering significant benefits. It has been found to reduce anxiety (Rainey, 2014) and depression (Hedberg et al., 2010), while also positively influencing the adoption of healthy behaviors (Hooker & Masters, 2016). Research even suggests that fostering a sense of purpose in life is an important aspect of preventive healthcare (Kim et al., 2014). When working with religious patients, it is important to recognize that they often bring a preexisting sense of identity to therapy. This religious identity can contribute to their overall sense of purpose and provide a foundation for exploring and addressing their therapeutic needs. By understanding and respecting the significance of their religious beliefs, therapists can effectively incorporate and build upon this existing sense of identity and purpose in the therapeutic journey.

All three elements, (1) a support system, (2) a positive outlook, and (3) a sense of purpose, are all beneficial within the therapeutic process. Salsman and colleagues (2005) conclude that two of the variables, social support and optimism offered through a patient's religiosity, have a positive impact on their psychological adjustment. While certain variables associated with the patient's faith may come up in therapy and seem to negatively impact them, a skillful therapist will shift the lens to these essential elements and utilize them in the therapeutic process to help those they are working with address their issues.

Conclusion

Sex therapy with religious patients can present significant challenges for therapists, requiring them to navigate diverse levels of diversity within and between different faith traditions. They must address conflicting messages related to sex, sexuality, and gender, while also confronting their own biases, all while prioritizing the best interests of the patient and maintaining respect for their religious beliefs. This task is far from easy. In some cases, the strong convictions held by the patient may seem to hinder the ability to offer solutions that address their specific concerns. It may be tempting to suggest that they leave their faith community as a solution to their problems. However, as discussed in this chapter, such suggestions are problematic given the significant influence and impact of religion on an individual's identity and interactions with others. Proposing that they abandon their faith or adopt another faith can be harmful and cause severe distress.

It is recommended that clinicians refrain from imposing their personal beliefs and attitudes about religion onto their patients. Exceptions are granted in cases involving spiritual, sexual, or psychological abuse, where intervention may be necessary. Even then, therapists must approach these delicate matters with skill and care to help the patient navigate through these challenges. Overall, clinicians should avoid automatically concluding that religion is a negative factor and strive to recognize the potential benefits it offers to the patient. Additionally, they should seek to integrate relevant elements of the patient's religious beliefs and practices into the therapeutic process.

Note

1 It should be noted that differences between collectivist and individual-istic tendencies do depend on the location of the faith group. For example, Sharabi (2018) argues that within the land of Israel, Jews take on a more individualistic mindset influenced by American culture, whereas Christians and Muslims within Israel are more collectivist. For the sake of this discussion, I am simply considering the theological framework and religious texts from which the religious tradition is based.

References

Bronfenbrenner, U. (2005). *Making Human Beings Human: Bioecological Perspectives on Human Development* (U. Bronfenbrenner, Ed.). Sage Publications.

Chandler, D., Sennott, S. L., & Constantinides, D. M. (2019). *Sex Therapy with Erotically Marginalized Clients: Nine Principles of Clinical Support.* Taylor & Francis Group.

Colwell, J., Pollard, A., & Pollard, A. (Eds.). (2015). *Readings for Reflective Teaching in Early Education.* Bloomsbury Academic.

Cook, J. A. (2021). *Worldview Theory, Whiteness, and the Future of Evangelical Faith.* Rowman & Littlefield Publishing Group.

Dashefsky, A. (1972). And the search goes on: The meaning of religio-ethnic identity and identification. *Sociological Analysis, 33*(4), 239–245. DOI: 10.2307/3710583

Fonseca, A., & Canavarro, M. C. (2020). Cognitive correlates of women's postpartum depression risk and symptoms: The contribution of dysfunctional beliefs and negative thoughts. *Journal of Mental Health*, *29*(6), 614–622. DOI: 10.1080/09638237.2019. 1581331

Friedman, S. (2019). Assessing and treating sexual dysfunctions in orthodox jewish couples: A Summary of 41 consecutive case. *Mental Health, Religion, & Culture*, *22*(9), 930–942. DOI:10.1080/136 74676.2019.1688269

Harandi, T. F., Taghinasab, M. M., & Nayeri, T. D. (2017). The correlation of social support with mental health: A meta-analysis. *Electron Physician*, *9*(9), 5212–5222. DOI: 10.19082/5212

Hedberg, P., Gustafson, Y., Alèx, L., & Brulin, C. (2010). Depression in relation to purpose in life among a very old population: A five-year follow-up study. *Aging & Mental Health*, *14*(6). DOI: 10.1080/13607861003713216

Holder, R. W., & Josephson, P. B. (2020). Donald Trump, white evangelicals, and 2020: A challenge for American pluralism. *Society (New Brunswick)*, *57*(5), 540–546. DOI: 10.1007/s12115–020–00525-z

Hooker, S. A., & Masters, K. S. (2016). Purpose in life is associated with physical activity measured by accelerometer. *Journal of Health Psychology*, *21*(6), 962–971. DOI: 10.1177/1359105314542822

Husen, T., & Postlethwaite, T. N. (Eds.). (1994). *International Encylopedia of Education* (2nd ed.). Pergamon/Elsevier Science.

Jacobson, C. (2023). *Abrahamic Faiths: Perspectives on Gender Identity and Sexuality* (2nd ed.). Scholars' Press.

Jacobson, C., & Hirt, K. (2021). *Handbook of Reading Theological German*. Zondervan Academic.

Kim, E. S., Strecher, V. J., & Ryff, C. D. (2014). Purpose in life and use of preventive health care services. *Psychological and Cognitive Sciences*, *111*(46), 16331–16336. DOI: 10.1073/pnas.141482611

Kim, H. S., Sherman, D. K., & Taylor, S. E. (2008). Culture and social support. *American Psychologist*, *63*(3), 518–526. DOI: 10.1037/0003–066X

Kitchen, J. A., Hallett, R. E., Perez, R. J., & Rivera, G. J. (2019). Advancing the use of ecological systems theory in college student research: The ecological systems interview tool. *Journal of College Student Development*, *60*(4), 381–400. DOI:10.1353/csd.2019.0043.

Laranjeira, C., & Querido, A. (2022). Hope and optimism as an opportunity to improve the "positive mental health" demand. *Frontiers in Psychology, 13*, 827320. DIO: 10.3389/fpsyg.2022.827320

Metz, J. B. (1990). Kirche nach Auschwitz. *Kirche und Israel, Neukirchener Theologische Zeitschrif, 5*, 99–108.

Miller, D. D. (2019). The mystery of evangelical Trump support? *Constellations, 26*(1), 43–58. DOI: 10.1111/1467–8675.12351

Mudryk, E. P., & Johnson, L. R. (2022). The impact of religiousness and beliefs about mental illness on help-seeking behaviors of Muslim Americans. *The Journal of Clinical Psychology, 79*(4), 1208–1222. DOI: 10.1002/jclp.23466

Myers, W. R. (2019). Following Trump: Are evangelicals willing participants in a "new" religion? *Theology today, 76*(2), 103–113. DOI: 10.1177/0040573619843893

Naeem, F., Sajid, S., Naz, S., & Phiri, P. (2023). Culturally adapted CBT – the evolution of psychotherapy adaptation frameworks and evidence. *The Cognitive Behaviour Therapist, 16*(10). DOI: 10.1017/S1754470X2300003X

Olszewska, I., Twardowska, A., & Katny, A. (Eds.). (2019). *Ashkenazim and Sephardim: Language Miscellanea*. Peter Lang.

Rainey, L. (2014). The Search for Purpose in life: An Exploration of Purpose, the Search Process, and Purpose Anxiety. [Masters]. University of Pennsylvania.

Reitsma, B. (2020). Don't curse the darkness, light a candle. The challenge of Islam within the culture diversity of Europe. *European Journal of Theology, 29*(1), 39–48. DOI: 10.5117/EJT2020.1.005.REIT

Reynolds, J., May, M., & Xian, H. (2019). Not by bread alone: Mobility experiences, religion, and optimism about future mobility. *Socius: Sociological Research for a Dynamic World, 5*, 1–15.

Salsman, J. M., Brown, T. L., Brechting, E. H., & Carlson, C. R. (2005). The link between religion and spirituality and psychological adjustment: The mediating role of optimism and social support. *Personality and Social Psychology Bulletin, 31*(4), 522–535. DOI: 10.1177/0146167204271563

Sethi, S., & Seligman, M. E. P. (1993). Optimism and fundamentalism. *Psychological Science, 4*(4), 256–259. DOI: 10.1111/j.1467–9280.1993.tb00271.x

Sharabi, M. (2018). Ethno-religious groups work values and ethics: the case of Jews, Muslims and Christians in Israel. *International Review of Sociology*, *28*(1), 171–192. DOI: 10.1080/03906701.2017.1385226

Shupe, A. D., & Stacey, W. A. (1982). *Born Again Politics and the Moral Majority: What Social Surveys Really Show*. Edwin Mellen Press.

Smart, J. (2019). *Disability Across the Developmental Lifespan: An Introduction for the Helping Professions* (J. Smart, Ed.). Springer Publishing Company.

Wafaa, E. Z., & Imad, M. (2022). How the Bronfenbrenner bio-ecological system theory explains the development of students' sense of belonging to school? *SAGE Open*, *12*(4), 215824402211340. DOI: 10.1177/21582440221134089

Warren, P., Van Eck, K., Townley, G., & Kloos, B. (2015). Relationships among religious coping, optimism, and outcomes for persons with psychiatric disabilities. *Psychology of Religion and Spirituality,*, *7*(2), 91–99. DOI: 10.1037/a0038346

2

The Problem with Sex Therapy

Introduction

Walking in the door, it was obvious by the way that they were dressed that they were a religious couple. As they sit down to begin the session, there is a feeling of hesitation in the room. Their demeanor exudes precariousness. The conversation is dismal. The assessment responses are painfully vague and the way they look at you almost feels hostile and untrusting. This is the scenario that all therapists dread. It leaves them feeling unprepared and uncertain of what direction to go in moving forward in the therapeutic process.

While this may be a nightmare scenario for many therapists, this initial assessment is already a positive outcome. The fact that this religious couple has come to therapy is something that should be celebrated. They recognize that they need help in some area of sexual concern, and they have come to treatment despite any misconception or hesitation that they may have about therapy in general and sex therapy specifically. In some instances, they have come despite the objection of their religious leader, who may completely reject the concept of therapy. You may ask yourself the question, why? Why would they reject therapeutic intervention when it can be helpful and even essential in a person's overall well-being? The answer is a bit complicated.

DOI: 10.4324/9781003242017-4

A Short History of the Relationship Between Psychology and Religion

It may be surprising to learn that the term "psychology" was coined by Phillip Melachton, a protégé of the Protestant Reformer Martin Luther (Rollins, 1999, 23). In its infancy, psychology was thought of as a branch of theology. The assertion still seems reasonable if considering a holistic approach to viewing an individual. It would not be until the nineteenth century that psychology as a scientific discipline began to emerge (Nevid, 2013, 5).

Yet, when it did emerge as a scientific discipline, the adversarial relationship against religion began almost immediately, almost as some form of sibling rivalry. Since the 1920's, the two subjects have been viewed as being in opposition to one another (Rollins & Ellens, 2004, 1). This opposition can be seen clearly in the writings of Sigmund Freud. In *Zwangshandlungen und Religionsübungen* (1907), he argues that religion and neurosis are similar. Twenty years later, he declares that religion is simply an illusion derived from human wishes (Freud, 1927, 39). Shortly after, John Dewey argued that religion was just a coping mechanism by providing a sense of security in a hazardous world (Dewey, 1929, 3). Carl Jung continued the attack on religion by labeling it the, "external problem" (Jung, 1938, 1).

There have been more direct attacks against particular religions as well. For example, there have been numerous articles and books written questioning the mental health of Jesus of Nazareth. One of the earliest examples is Oskar Panizza, who described Jesus as psychopathological and paranoid (Panizza, 1898). Publications on the topic were plentiful enough that Albert Schweitzer was able to write his third doctoral dissertation examining assertions made by psychologists concerning the mental health of Jesus of Nazareth (Schweitzer, 1913).

As one might envision, when confronted with such adversarial stances, the responding parties often reciprocate in a similar manner. It is not infrequent to encounter reports from patients wherein their spiritual leaders have openly criticized or opposed psychological services. These actions, whether initiated by mental health practitioners or religious authorities, invariably result in the underutilization of vital mental health services within religious communities, thereby perpetuating a significant gap in access to comprehensive care.

Recent research shows that within all three Abrahamic faith traditions, members are hesitant about seeking mental health services. It has long been held that within the Orthodox Jewish community, members are reluctant to seek treatment for mental illness (Pirutinsky & Rosmarin, 2022). In many evangelical Christian communities, mental illness is believed to be the product of spiritual causes, thus, many evangelicals find it unnecessary to seek therapeutic intervention (Lloyd et al., 2022). Likewise, recent research shows how underutilized mental health services are in Muslim communities as well (Ali et al., 2022).

While this may be upsetting to learn that spiritual leaders have taken negative stances against therapy, should it *really* be surprising? Have sex therapists not also taken negative stances against religion?

For decades now, it has been known that scientists are less religious than the general population and that among the scientific community, psychologists are the least religious among scientists (Argyle & Beit-Hallahmi, 1975). Additionally, Turner and Stayton (2022) state that some view sexuality and spirituality as sworn adversaries. Therefore, it is easy to reason that therapists working in areas of human sexuality often have negative views of religion. This could come from their own cognitive reasoning, life experiences, or any number of additional factors. Nevertheless, it is not uncommon to learn that a sex therapist has somehow been inspired to enter the field due to negative experiences in their past that intersect sexuality and religion.

While we all have life experiences that bring us to where we are presently, we must be careful about how those experiences manifest in the work that we do. Despite any negative experiences that the clinician has personally had in the past, research does indicate the benefits of including religion and spirituality in the therapeutic relationship (Dein, 2018). Yet despite this, there is often a transferential and countertransferential element that manifests, which is very dangerous to the patient (Abernethy & Lancia, 1998).

When understanding the often turbulent relationship that psychology and religion have, clinicians should be extra mindful when working with religious individuals and couples. The step to therapy is often difficult for people of faith, especially when they are coming to discuss sexual issues, which are often seen as taboo to practice and inappropriate even in conversation. There are many fears and biases that they must overcome. For example, a recent study shows that conservatives fear that non-Christian identifying therapists would be dismissive or even ridicule their religious beliefs. The study also reported that there was a fear of being exposed to antireligious beliefs and that the therapist would give recommendations or suggest behavioral changes that could contradict their religious beliefs or be immoral (Salem & Hijazi, 2019). Unfortunately, some of these fears are not left unwarranted, especially when it comes to clinician's bias concerning religiously informed boundaries around sex, sexuality, and gender.

Appreciating and Respecting Boundaries

Far too often, the way that a religious patient thinks about sex is viewed as sex-negative by sex therapists and sex educators. While it may be true that the religious patient holds more conservative and less permissive ideas about sex, sexuality, and gender, it does not necessarily mean that they are sex-negative. What it does mean is that they have religiously informed boundaries around sex. These boundaries should be respected by the clinician.

It is interesting to notice how therapists encourage patients to have boundaries in all areas of their lives, and yet it has been observed that many of these same therapists find issues when patients have religiously informed boundaries that involve prohibitions against certain sexual behavior. However, boundaries are healthy in all relationships – including sexual ones. For many religious people, their religiously informed boundaries are empowering to both them and their relationships. As such, sex therapists should offer the same judgment-free environment that they offer to patients from diverse sexual backgrounds and expressions.

From my experience, the problematic factor is normally not the boundaries that the person holds about sex. Nor is it necessarily the teaching that their faith has concerning the issues related to sex, sexuality, and gender. Most often, the issues stem from the way that the community, under the leadership of their religious authority, reacts and responds to these topics and the atmosphere that they create. There are two ways that this commonly manifests itself within religious communities, I refer to them as **Community Gossip** and **Community Discipline**.

Community Gossip

Often in highly structured, highly regulated communities, there is the tendency for a person to compare themselves to others or judge themself based on others. There is also the tendency to find faults in others in order to deflect attention from oneself. It is not uncommon to see people within a religious community revert to the kindergarten tactic of telling the religious leader what other people in the community are doing wrong.

This, of course, causes several major problems. First, it creates an unsafe environment where people feel that they must be on guard and are unable to be open and authentic around others. Their life often becomes a facade and many times, they feel they are living a lie or having to perform in front of others. The second major issue is that it creates a cycle effect where people feel that they should tell on someone before someone tells on them.

In both of these scenarios, people live in a constant state of fear, wondering if someone is talking about them, either to others in their religious community, to the clergy, or wondering if someone is ever going to discover the double life that they are being forced to live since they cannot live authentically within their community. These feelings have a high emotional impact. They affect a person's view of themselves, their religious community, and religion in general. Yet the phenomenon of this behavior is not a tenant of any of the Abrahamic faiths, nor is it part of sacred texts.

Community Discipline

Within Christianity, it is not uncommon to learn that someone has been the subject of community discipline when they have violated the guidelines and principles of that community. What the discipline actually entails really depends upon the individual community. For some, the discipline could be as simple as reciting a prayer. For others, they could be required to stand up in front of the entire congregation, confess their sins, and ask for forgiveness. Still, others can be more extreme. Instances have been recorded where people have been forced to sit on the back pew of the congregation alone, while others in the community have been instructed not to communicate or talk to the individual until the punishment period was over, and even instances where physical punishment was given.

Disciplinary actions in themselves are not bad. Even professional organizations for psychologists and sex therapists have disciplinary actions when a member violates certain rules of membership. However, when the disciplinary action goes beyond trying to help the member and instead tries to embarrass, degrade, or hurt the member, the action moves from disciplinary to abusive.

It should be noted that while none of these disciplinary scenarios are rooted in sacred texts, there are those who still try to justify and base their unjust actions on biblical texts. Therefore, it is not uncommon that a person will believe that their unjust actions, or the unjust action of someone else, is justified. This is similar to the justification of any abusive behavior by an abused individual. However, a clear distinction must once again be made between boundaries and abuse.

Boundaries, regardless of how restrictive the clinician may find them, can be very good. Let's take, for example, the boundary against premarital sex that many religious people hold. While this may seem sex negative or potentially problematic, it could be very empowering for a person of faith. Perhaps the individual does not feel prepared to have conversations and discussions about sexual interaction with their partner. This boundary eliminates the need to have such conversations until they feel they are more equipped. Refraining from sex until marriage may also provide them with peace of mind by not having to worry about pregnancies or possible sexually transmitted infections, both of which are realistic risks associated with sexual interaction.

What may be an empowering boundary for some can be traumatic for others. Suppose someone decides not to keep the boundary concerning premarital sex and engages in sexual relations. Perhaps they decided not to keep the boundary because they have no personal conviction about such behavior. However, due to the community gossip, as mentioned above, people in the community start telling others in the community about their personal decisions and the choice that they made to be sexually active. It is not uncommon to hear it phrased that the person "fell into sin" or has become "**backslidden**." At this stage, the person who decides not to keep the religiously informed boundary may feel socially ostracized and begin feeling guilt and shame based on communal expectations.

The situation can become more problematic with the addition of out-of-control spiritual authority. As mentioned, there are instances where spiritual discipline includes physical and psychological punishments and abuse. Primarily, public humiliation and isolation are most often used. It should be noted that in some religious communities, breaching certain rules for membership disqualifies a member from participating in certain official community positions. For example, within a church, if a person engages in premarital sex, they may not be allowed to teach Sunday School or play guitar in the Praise Team. Such actions, in general, should not be considered abuse but part of the autonomy of the community to uphold their religious convictions. In this instance, no one is physically, emotionally, or psychologically harmed, though they may be a bit disappointed that they can no longer participate at the level they previously were.

Additionally, there is a third scenario wherein the person of faith has strong convictions concerning premarital sex and has chosen to maintain this religiously informed boundary. However, at some point, they are involved in a relationship that becomes sexually involved. The person feels guilt and shame over their sexual decision-making and has difficulty finding congruence between what they believe and the way that they acted sexually. In this scenario, the person is not the subject of spiritual abuse and despite the distress they are currently experiencing, it is not an indication that their religious teachings are dangerous or harmful.

In such instances, clinicians need to be respectful of the patient's decision to maintain religiously informed boundaries. They should not try to convince the patient to alter their conviction or leave their religion. By respecting the patient's conviction, the clinician is able to engage in conversation to understand why specific boundaries are important to them. Additionally, it provides clarity to the patient about their own thoughts and beliefs concerning their religious convictions and why they choose to hold them. Such exploration can also provide an understanding of why they acted out of alignment with their boundaries.

Assessing Patient's Level of Religious Observance

With the amount of diversity found within a religious community, understanding all the nuances of a particular religion would be difficult, if not impossible, to achieve. It is also important to recognize that each person may have a different level of religious observance despite the level of orthodoxy their religious community holds to. Most religiously identifiable persons can be categorized into one of four stages:

1. observant;
2. moderately observant;
3. low observance; and
4. non-observant.

Understanding which of these stages the patient may be in is essential in providing them the best possible care. Determining where the patient may be is as simple as asking. I recommend asking a question such as:

◆ *So, if you don't mind me asking, how would you define your level of religious observance?*

While such questions may seem awkward to ask at first, they are key to working with religious patients since competency within a faith tradition is impossible due to the amount of diversity present. Likewise, even if you have experience working with a particular faith group, it is always in the therapist's best interest to ask for clarity concerning theological terms and positions to fully understand the patient's level of religious observance and gain insight into their thoughts concerning a specific topic or issue.

The clinician should never feel inadequate for not fully understanding their patient's religious beliefs concerning sexual issues. Remember, if the patient was seeking theological clarification, they would have talked to their clergy. While you need to be aware of theological concepts, you are not required or expected to know all of the nuances found between and within faith traditions.

Gaining The Patient's Confidence

Due to the rocky past between psychology and religion, it is not uncommon for religious patients to come to therapy with reservations and hesitation, the same as would be expected by marginalized groups. It is the clinician's responsibility to aid in overcoming the patient's reservations. There are five principles that can be very useful in achieving this goal, (1) establishing confidentiality, (2) being inquisitive, (3) distinguishing between cultural competency, cultural awareness, and cultural responsiveness, (4) adopting the patient's language, and (5) avoiding negative comments.

Establishing Confidentiality

Confidentiality is exceptionally important to religious patients, especially when dealing with sensitive topics related to sex, sexuality, and gender. This is supported by the findings of a recent study that noted that Muslim women highly valued confidentiality above all else in the therapeutic relationship (Grey et al., 2020). It is therefore suggested that clinicians work to establish confidentiality in early communication with the patient.

Often this will be included in my opening remarks during the initial assessment, although it may take place even earlier during telephone or email communications. Typically, a simple statement assuring confidentiality can be made in opening remarks. Such as:

- ◆ *I'm really happy to work with you and want you to know that everything we discuss is confidential.*
- ◆ *As we get started, I want to assure you that everything we talk about is private and stays between us.*

At the close of the initial session, it is also good to reiterate the confidential nature of the services by saying:

- ◆ *I am really looking forward to working with you and I want to remind you that anything we discuss in our time together is confidential and will stay between us.*

It should go without saying that certain caveats need to be included based on the location of services provided and the governing laws of the area. Being upfront concerning issues related to mandatory reporting, for example, helps the patient build trust in the clinician's forthrightness and honesty early on.

Being Inquisitive

As mentioned in the previous chapter, religion and spirituality have a positive impact on a person's physical and mental health. The impact is so great that some argue for the inclusion of religious resources in hospitals, including healthcare providers inquiring about religious and spiritual issues (Gad et al., 2022). Thus, it is important for clinicians to be inquisitive concerning the spiritual life and religious beliefs of those that they provided services to. It is recommended that clinicians include questions concerning religion in their intake and assessment forms.

Some possible questions to include could be:

- ◆ *What is your religious background?*
- ◆ *What role does religion and/or spirituality have in your life?*

◆ *Do you have positive or negative feelings toward religion/spirituality?*

◆ *If you hold any religious/spiritual practices currently, are they the same or different from those you grew up with?*

Each of these questions offers the clinician the chance to ask further follow-up questions. Such questions can lead to discovering past religious trauma or that the patient is deeply religious and observant. This also gives the clinician the chance to understand the particular faith tradition, level of observance, and religiously informed ideas concerning sex, sexuality, and gender that they may have. This is an important intersection of dialogue that can greatly aid in further developing discussion and intervention later in the therapeutic process.

Distinguishing Between Cultural Competency, Cultural Awareness, and Cultural Responsiveness

Much has been written about the importance of cultural competency. It is defined as the "ability to engage effectively with individuals of diverse cultural backgrounds" (Soto et al., 2021). The idea is that by understanding the patient's culture, the clinician will better understand the patient – their way of thought, behavior, and motivation. Yet, it has been pointed out that cultural competency is something that is not actually obtainable. To highlight this point, we can remember that Islam is the most ethnically diverse religion in the world. With each set of believers having distinct identities, beliefs, and customs, all of which are based on their geographic location. How can one therapist ever expect to gain competency?

What a therapist can be conscious of is cultural awareness. We can be aware that there are both major differences and subtle nuances within any faith tradition. We can aim to be respectful of the patient's unique beliefs within their faith tradition while observing how complex and complicated many of these concepts actually are. We can also be mindful of our own biases that arise when those we serve willingly open up and share important aspects of their faith with us.

To do this effectively, Johnson and Vasquez (2022) showcase three qualities important in demonstrating cultural awareness,

(1) cultural sensitivity, (2) cultural knowledge, and (3) cultural empathy. **Cultural sensitivity** is defined as respect for and knowledge of culturally diverse people. The term **cultural knowledge** refers to actual facts about a particular culture and knowledge about the diversity within and between cultures. This quality can be gained from books, courses, and other educational materials. Finally, **cultural empathy** is the ability to relate to someone's cultural worldview. Cultural empathy is gained through increased exposure and shared experiences with people from a diverse culture (Johnson & Vasquez, 2022, 46).

Cultural awareness can then be put into therapeutic practice through **cultural responsiveness**, the adapting of therapeutic treatment in response to the patient's culture, religious, or spiritual observance. Recently, de Abreu Costa and Moreira-Almeida (2022) demonstrated ways to adapt cognitive behavioral therapy with respect to patient's religious beliefs. Additionally, current research also suggests that therapists would benefit from both training and supervision in working with a culturally diverse population to better understand how to adapt treatment in an effective way (Mathieson et al., 2023).

Adopting the patient's Language

Within any culture, there is specific language that is commonly understood within that population. This is also true with religious traditions and the language and lingo changes based on the specific faith community. In Chapters 4–6 of this book, some terms specific to sex, sexuality, and gender as they relate to Judaism, Christianity, and Islam are given; however, it is important for the therapist to build a more comprehensive faith vocabulary. In the early stages of working with patients, this language is easily attained simply by asking the patient what particular terms mean. In order to avoid sounding ill-prepared or not competent, questions can be phrased in a way that seeks specifics from the patient, like in the following example:

◆ *You have used the word _____ several times. Tell me what that means to you specifically.*

With many marginalized groups, it is important to use the particular vernacular, languages, words, metaphors, etc., of that group (Chandler et al., 2019). By doing such, you help the patient feel more at ease and you are able to gain greater insight into their cognition through psycholinguistics (Kambara et al., 2020; Clackson et al., 2022).

Avoiding negative comments.

It can become very easy to fall into the habit of repeating a patient's negative thoughts and feelings about religion when trying to relate to a patient and adopt the language that they're using. For example, if a patient mentions that their boss said something inappropriate to them at work, it could feel very natural to agree with them and comment that their boss's behavior was wrong. Yet, this is something that you do not want to do when it comes to their religious beliefs, as it could interfere with the therapeutic alliance by strengthening fears and biases that the patient may already have.

Since there is often a perceived divide between psychological services and religious communities, by agreeing with or even repeating the patient's negative comments about their religious beliefs, it can serve to solidify cognitions about psychological services that they may have, and cause them to be defensive. While it is the patient's right to say negative things about the communities that they are a part of and the faith tradition that they hold, it is never alright for the therapist to do the same. Due to the sensitive nature of this matter, it is recommended that when a patient brings up negative topics, the therapist simply listens or asks follow-up questions like the following:

- *You said your pastor called you out in front of the congregation, what exactly does that mean?*
- *You mentioned that no one in your community is allowed to talk to you, what is that reality like?*
- *Since you're forbidden from participating in religious activities, what will you do now?*

These questions allow the patient to continue to discuss and process what is transpiring without feeling judged by the therapist and becoming defensive. By exercising restraint in this area, the clinician can demonstrate that they are without bias in working with people of faith and truly offer a judgment-free environment. When such behavior is demonstrated, the patient is much more likely to open up and be willing to provide more detailed disclosure that propels the therapeutic journey further.

The Use of the Term Client vs. Patient

The term "client" is often preferred by many practitioners to refer to individuals in a therapeutic alliance, as opposed to the traditional term "patient." This shift in terminology was popularized by Carl Rogers in his seminal work, Client-Centered Therapy: Its Current Practice, Implications, and Theory, initially published in 1951 (Rogers, 2003). It is noteworthy that Rogers embarked on his academic journey studying theology before transitioning to psychology (Hough & Tassoni, 2021, 150). His exploration of the self and the organismic self, both of which possess theological roots, highlights the influence of theology in his conceptual framework. By using the term "client," practitioners acknowledge the importance of empowering individuals in the therapeutic process and fostering a collaborative relationship based on respect, autonomy, and self-discovery.

However, in line with the title of this book, I choose to use the term "patient" instead. While this might come as a surprise to some readers, I believe that the term "patient" is more suitable, particularly when working with religious individuals and couples.

1. Let us first begin by considering a quick etymological point. Neuberger (1999) rightly explains that "Patient comes from the Latin 'patiens,' from 'patior,' to suffer or bear." The term "client," on the other hand, comes from the Latin word "cliens" and is synonymous with "customer" or "patron" (Shevell, 2009). We first must begin

by asking: what is the role of the sex therapist? To help someone who has something difficult to bear and is perhaps suffering? Or is it strictly a business interaction?

2. Second, consider the importance that the use of words has on the therapeutic relationship, on the part of the provider and the one being served. Fuks (2021, 17–22) demonstrates that words and language have an influence on the clinical interaction between the patient and doctor. By using the term "patient," a specific framework and system is already in place with pre-established roles and responsibilities. Thus the relationship takes on a more serious arrangement. Additionally, in the UK, it was found that the use of the word "client" within the field of social work introduced a hierarchical power position, wherein a "good" client was one who would listen to the social worker without question. And those receiving help were given labels such as "deserving" and "undeserving poor" (McLaughlin, 2009).

3. A third point of consideration is the misconception that the term "client" conjures. Since the term is connected with consumerism, it adds to the common narrative and misconceptions within sex therapy. Many are still confused and uncertain as to what actually transpires within the profession. Some even assume that some type of sexual service or activity takes place between the therapist and the "client." These misconceptions are reinforced by the use of the term "client," since the term "client" is often commonly used within sex work to refer to the person who is buying the sexual service.

4. For those who are religious and already struggle with their decision to seek psychotherapy and discuss sexual issues, the use of the term "patient" to refer to them helps to solidify the legitimacy and the clinical aspect of the work that is being done.

5. While it may be common practice to use the word "client" as opposed to "patient," please take into consideration the preference of those actually being served. Research on the subject has been conducted. In 2005, a study that

compared the label "patient" with that of "survivor" among those who had breast or prostate cancer, showed that among college students, the term "survivor" was favored because of what they thought it said about the person who had battled cancer. Yet, ironically enough, those who had survived cancer preferred the use of the term "patient" (Deber et al., 2005). Additionally, studies have since been conducted yielding similar results.

Language is important. The language that we use sets the parameters for the work that we do as psychotherapists. That language is interpreted by those we serve in the way that they understand the role of the clinician and their role as the patient. In essence, it sets the framework for the entire therapeutic relationship. As such, we, as clinicians, should be mindful of the terminology we use, the impact it has on those we serve, and the impact it has on our work. It seems difficult to deny that the use of the term "patient" is far more fitting and adds to the legitimacy of the work that we do.

Conclusion

That chapter demonstrates that sex therapy with religious individuals and couples presents unique challenges for therapists, necessitating a careful and nuanced approach. The historical relationship between psychology and religion has often been adversarial, with Freudian theories and subsequent criticisms contributing to a perceived conflict between the two domains. Religious communities, influenced by these tensions, may be skeptical of or even opposed to seeking therapeutic intervention, which can result in the underutilization of mental health services. On the other hand, therapists working in the field of human sexuality may harbor negative views toward religion due to personal experiences or cognitive reasoning.

However, it is crucial for therapists to approach the therapeutic process with an open mind and a willingness to understand and respect the religious beliefs and boundaries of their patients. The journey towards seeking therapy for religious individuals and couples is often a difficult one, as they may feel conflicted between their faith teachings and the need for help in addressing sexual concerns. Thus, their initial hesitation should not be seen as reluctance to therapy itself but rather as an internal struggle to reconcile their faith with the challenges they face.

Therapists should consider that religiously informed boundaries around sex, sexuality, and gender are not necessarily indicative of a negative or repressive attitude toward these topics. Rather, these boundaries are often empowering for individuals and contribute to the well-being of their relationships. Just as therapists encourage boundaries in other aspects of their patient's lives, they should extend the same respect and non-judgmental attitude towards religiously informed boundaries.

Understanding the diverse levels of religious observance within a community is also vital. Therapists should not feel inadequate for not fully grasping the nuances of every faith tradition. Instead, they should focus on creating a safe and confidential space where patients feel comfortable sharing their beliefs and experiences. Inquiring about patients' spiritual lives and religious beliefs, as well as embracing cultural competency, can further enhance the therapeutic alliance and facilitate meaningful progress.

It is essential for therapists to shed their own biases and negative experiences related to religion, recognizing that spirituality and religion can play a positive role in a person's overall well-being. Research has shown the benefits of incorporating religion and spirituality into therapy, and therapists should be mindful of avoiding negative comments or imposing their own beliefs on their patients. By embracing these principles, therapists can build trust, instill confidence, and guide religious patients toward positive change in their sexual lives and relationships.

Ultimately sex therapy with religious individuals and couples requires therapists to navigate the complexities and sensitivities surrounding faith, sexuality, and therapy. By fostering a respectful and inclusive therapeutic environment, therapists can support their patients in reconciling their religious beliefs with their sexual concerns and, ultimately, contribute to their overall sexual and relational well-being.

References

Abernethy, A. D., & Lancia, J. J. (1998). Religion and the psychotherapeutic relationship: Transferential and countertransferential dimensions. *The Journal of Psychotherapy Practice and Research*, *7*(4), 281–289.

Ali, S., Elsayed, D., Elahi, S., Zai, B., & Awaad, R. (2022). Predicting rejection attitudes toward utilizing formal mental health services in Muslim women in the US: Results from the Muslims' perceptions and attitudes to mental health study. *International Journal of Social Psychiatry*, *68*(3), 662–669. DOI: 10.1177/00207640211001084

Argyle, M., & Beit-Hallahmi, B. (1975). *The Social Psychology of Religion*. Routledge and Kegan Paul.

Chandler, D., Sennott, S., & Constantinides, D. (2019). *Sex Therapy with Erotically Marginalized Clients: Nine Principles of Clinical Support*. Routledge.

Clackson, K., Pohran, N., Galli, R. M., Labno, L., Farias, M., Bekinschtein, T. A., & Noreika, V. (2022). Cambridge psycholinguistic inventory of christian beliefs: A registered report of construct validity, internal consistency and test–retest reliability. *Behavior Research Methods*, *54*(1), 457–474. DOI: 10.3758/s13428-021-01632-3

de Abreu Costa, M., & Moreira-Almeida, A. (2022). Religion-adapted cognitive behavioral therapy: A review and description of techniques. *Journal of Religion and Health*, *61*(1), 443–466. DOI: 10.1007/s10943–021–01345-z

Deber, R. B., Kraetschmer, N., Urowitz, S., & Sharpe, N. (2005). Patient, consumer, client, or customer: What do people want to be called? *Health Expectations*, *8*(4), 345–351.

Dein, S. (2018). Against the stream: Religion and mental health – the case for the inclusion of religion and spirituality into psychiatric care. *BJPsych Bulletin*, *42*(3), 127–129. DOI: 10.1192/bjb.2017.13

Dewey, J. (1929). *The Quest for Certainty: A Study of the Relation of Knowledge and Action*. Minton, Balch, and Company.

Freud, S. (1927). *Die Zukunft einer Illusion*. Internationaler Psycho-analytischer Verlag.

Fuks, A. (2021). *The Language of Medicine*. Oxford University Press.

Gad, I., Tan, X.-W. C., Williams, S., Itawi, S., Dahbour, L., Rotter, Z., Mitro, G., Rusch, C., Perkins, S., & Ali, I. (2022). The religious and spiritual needs of patients in the hospital setting do not depend on patient level of religious/spiritual observance and should be initiated by healthcare providers. *Journal of Religion and Health*, *61*, 1120–1138. DOI: 10.1007/s10943-020-01103-7

Grey, I., Tohme, P., Thomas, J., Mazrouie, M. A., & Abi-Habib, R. (2020). Preferred therapist characteristics of muslim college women in the united arab emirates: Implications for psychotherapy. *Mental Health, Religion & Culture*, *23*(9), 745–755. DOI: 10.1080/13674676.2020.1795823

Hough, M., & Tassoni, P. (2021). *Counselling Skills and Theory*, 5th edition. Hodder Education.

Johnson, J. D., & Vasquez, M. J. T. (2022). *Multicultural Therapy: A Practice Imperative*. American Psychological Association.

Jung, C. G. (1938). *Psychology and Religion*. Yale University Press.

Kambara, T., Umemura, T., Ackert, M., & Yang, Y. (2020). The relationship between psycholinguistic features of religious words and core dimensions of religiosity: A survey study with Japanese participants. *Religions*, *11*(12), 673. DOI: 10.3390/rel11120673

Lloyd, C. E.M., Mengistu, B. S., & Reid, G. (2022). "His main problem was not being in a relationship with God": Perceptions of depression, help-seeking, and treatment in evangelical Christianity. *Frontiers in Psychology*, *13*, 831534. DOI: 10.3389/fpsyg.2022.831534

Mathieson, F., Garrett, S., Stubbe, M., Hilder, J., Tester, R., Fedchuck, D., Dunlop, A., & Dowell, A. (2023). Therapist voices on a youth mental health pilot: Responsiveness to diversity and therapy modality. *International Journal of Environmental Research and Public Health*, *20*(3), 1834. DOI: 10.3390/ijerph20031834

McLaughlin, H. (2009). What's in a name: "client", "patient", "customer", "consumer", "expert by experience", "service user" – what's next? *The British Journal of Social Work*, *39*(6), 1101–1117.

Neuberger, J. (1999). Do we need a new word for patients? Lets do away with "patients". *BMJ*, *318*(7200), 1756–1757. DOI: 10.1136/bmj.318.7200.1756

Nevid, J. S. (2013). *Psychology: Concepts and Applications*. Cengage Learning.

Panizza, O. (1898). Christus in psicho-patologischer Beleuchtung. *Zürcher Diskuszjonen*, *5*(1), 1–8.

Pirutinsky, S., & Rosmarin, D. H. (2022). A comparative study of mental health diagnoses, symptoms, treatment, and medication use among Orthodox Jews. *Transcultural Psychiatry*, *59*(6), 756–766. DOI: 10.1177/13634615211068607

Rogers, C. R. (2003). *Client-centered Therapy: Its Current Practice, Implications and Theory*. Constable.

Rollins, W. G. (1999). *Soul and Psyche: The Bible in Psychological Perspective*. Fortress Press.

Rollins, W. G., & Ellens, J. H. (Eds.). (2004). *Psychology and the Bible: From Freud to Kohut*. Praeger.

Salem, S., & Hijazi, A. (2019). Does therapist–rater religious match predict higher therapist ratings? *Counseling and values*, *64*(1), 90–107. DOI: 10.1002/cvj.12096

Schweitzer, A. (1913). *Die psychiatrische Beurteilung Jesu: Darstellung und Kritik*. Mohr.

Shevell, M. I. (2009). What do we call "them"? The "patient" versus "client" dichotomy. *Developmental Medicine & Child Neurology*, *51*(10), 770–772. DOI: 10.1111/j.1469–8749.2009.03304.x

Soto, J. A., Mena, J. A., Borge, M., Borge, M. R., Witherspoon, D. P., & Dawson-Andoh, N. A. (2021). Multicultural competence building blocks: Multicultural psychology courses promote multicultural knowledge and ethnic identity. *Teaching of Psychology*. DOI: 10.1177/00986283211031854

Turner, G. W., & Stayton, W. R. (2022). Are sex therapy and God, strange bedfellows? Case studies illuminating the intersection of client sexuality with spirituality, religion, faith or belief practices. *Sexual and Relationship Therapy*, *37*(3), 324–341. DOI: 10.1080/14681994.2021.2007235

3

The Protocol

Introduction

Working with a new demographic can be a daunting experience for even the most experienced therapists. It's natural to want to project confidence and insightfulness during therapy sessions while also creating a safe space for patients to open up. This can be particularly challenging when patients are skeptical or cautious of the therapeutic process. This can leave even the most skilled and astute therapist feeling overwhelmed, anxious, and unsure of their direction. Establishing a proper protocol is essential to navigate these scenarios, ensuring that therapists feel equipped and confident as they guide their patients through the therapeutic process.

There is little doubt that the vast majority of sex therapists have experience with the PLISSIT model. Jack S. Annon first introduced the PLISSIT model in 1976 (Annon, 1976). Since that time, there have been numerous studies demonstrating the efficacy of the model, and despite how long the model has been around, it is still referenced in even the most recent peer-reviewed studies (Rash et al., 2023). PLISSIT is an acronym for **P**ermission, **L**imited **I**nformation, **S**pecific **S**uggestions, & **I**ntensive **T**herapy. This model should be thought of as the framework in which sex therapy with religious patients is conducted. It is within this framework that the protocol will be fulfilled.

DOI: 10.4324/9781003242017-5

For some, it is helpful to imagine the PLISSIT model as steps in the therapeutic journey. However, steps indicate a linear progression, which is not always the case within therapy. Personally, I envision therapy as a process that is always in motion, similar to a wheel that is turning. So I suggest imagining the PLISSIT model as demonstrated in Figure 3.1. The figure shows a circular image that includes Limited Information, Specific Suggestions, and Intensive Therapy on the outer circumference. At the center of this figure is Permission, highlighting its relevance and constant inclusion in all of the different parts of this model.

The first step in sex therapy with religious patients is always Permission. This step is essential and should be part of your intake process. This is not only the time to ask the patients if they are okay with you talking about sex, but this is the time that they can give themselves permission to discuss sexual issues. I usually begin the discussion like this:

◆ *As we start, I want to first get your permission. A lot of the things that we are going to discuss are sexual and I know that makes many people uncomfortable because it can feel difficult or awkward sharing personal and intimate aspects of our lives – are you okay with me talking about these things?*

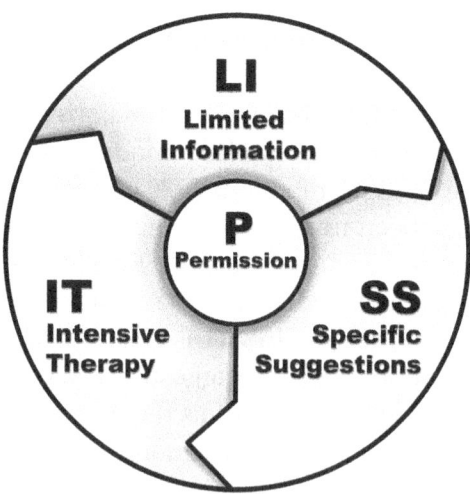

FIGURE 3.1 The PLISSIT Model.

While gaining this permission is ethically important in preparing the patient for sex therapy, for the religious patient, it can be even more essential for them to give themselves permission to discuss these topics, as even discussing them can be seen as taboo and, in some cases, sinful. So many of my patients never discussed sex openly before coming to therapy because they have been told it is wrong or that they shouldn't do it. So, I tell them:

♦ *I also want you to give yourself permission. I know it may not feel comfortable at first, especially when you're not used to talking about sex openly, but during our time together, will you give yourself permission to discuss these things?*

It should not be underestimated how deeply profound it is for religious patients to give themselves permission to discuss sex openly. Many have never done so, not even with their partners, regardless of how long they have been married. It should never be assumed that because a patient is coming to sex therapy they realize they will need to discuss personal sexual issues. It is possible that a person comes seeking help for sexual problems without realizing the need to disclose sexual details. Having such discussions about sex can feel "wrong" or "inappropriate," regardless of the context. Therefore, when patients give themselves permission to discuss sex, it is very freeing and allows them to express thoughts and feelings that they have previously suppressed.

The other three components of the PLISSIT model can be divided into two categories: (1) short-term intervention, consisting of limited information and specific suggestions, and (2) long-term intervention, consisting of intensive therapy.

When it comes to Limited Information, this part of the process should be thought of as the educational component of the therapeutic process. Within the practice of sex therapy, psychosexual education is often required; with religious patients, it's paramount. Many religious patients have had little to no sex education. Providing sex education may be required throughout the entire therapeutic relationship; however, it will be an essential component of the early stages of the therapeutic process.

While providing basic sex education may seem trivial to experienced clinicians, there are benefits to a religious patient's lack of sex education. The only thing worse than no sex education is bad sex education. It is far too common that a therapist must aid their patients in unlearning unhelpful attitudes, beliefs, and general misinformation about sex. However, the advantage of the patient having zero sex education is that they do not have to spend time unlearning incorrect information. There are plenty of misconceptions that all patients, religious or not, will have based on things they have seen in the media, learned from friends and family, and picked up from previous relationships. Religious patients will have the addition of what they have heard in their religious communities or the way they have interpreted religious texts dealing with sexual issues.

When offering patients Specific Suggestions to help address their presenting problem, it is important to remember the patient's religious background. For example, it may be easy to suggest that a female patient struggling with anorgasmia try using a vibrator, since they are shown to be effective in helping women achieve orgasm (Dubinskaya et al., 2023). This suggestion would be problematic, though, when dealing with women of certain faith traditions. Therefore, we must be cautious never to suggest something that is counter to the patient's religious beliefs and convictions. Doing so will negatively impact the patient-clinician relationship.

The final part of the PLISSIT model is Intensive Therapy. This is where the clinician can help the patient in dealing with deeper psychological and emotional factors that impact their sexual functioning. When working with religious patients, it is often the case that issues related to their religious community are brought up by the patient. This is most likely the time when the clinician could have the strongest reaction to what the patient is telling them. It is also the time that the clinician must exercise the highest professional ethics and check their personal biases that could hinder the therapeutic process.

Please notice that both brief therapy techniques and intensive therapy are required when working with religious patients. I call this a two-tiered approach to therapy. The brief therapy techniques will help to reduce the anxiety that the patient has concerning their immediate or surface-level issue. This reduction in anxiety is essential before most patients will be able to move into more intensive therapy. Seeing early results from the brief therapy stage also motivates the patients to dive into deeper therapeutic work.

From the Framework to the Actual Work

Now that the framework for how the therapeutic process will operate has been established let's look at the specific protocol that should be used when working with religious patients. The protocol has four specific steps.

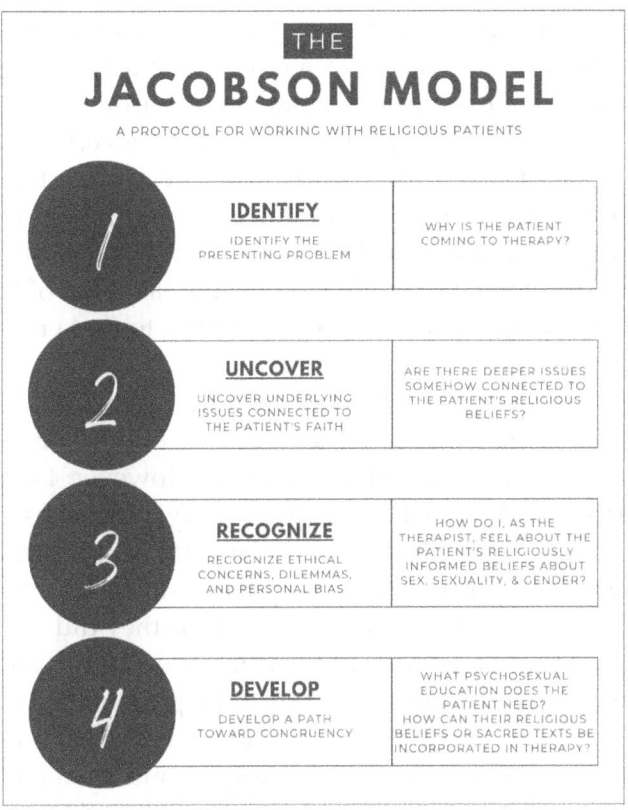

FIGURE 3.2 The Jacobson Model.

Step One – Identify

The first step when working with a religious patient should be the same step when working with any patient – **identify** the presenting problem. Why is the patient coming to therapy? More specifically, why are they coming to sex therapy? For religious patients, some of the most common issues are unconsummated marriages, sexual pain, ejaculatory issues, and issues related to sexual orientation. Guilt and shame, as you may imagine, also are common themes, though one should be careful not to automatically assume that the guilt and shame come directly from the religious beliefs themselves, though they could still be connected.

For example, suppose a patient comes to therapy because they feel guilt and shame about having sex outside of marriage. Their cognitions concerning premarital sex have been informed by their religious beliefs. Thus, the guilt and shame that they are experiencing is directly linked to their religious beliefs and/or community. It should, however, also be noted that many patients who are not religious feel guilt and shame around sex as well. While it may be easy to point to and identify certain religious teachings or ideas as the culprit, it is the easiest target. The truth is that guilt and shame around sex are common in almost all cultures, regardless of the presence or absence of religion. Therefore, the clinician should not take the easy shot of attacking the patient's religion and instead be willing to find creative and helpful resolutions.

As a side note, guilt and shame are not always bad. Sometimes in an effort to be extremely "sex positive," clinicians desire to eradicate and erase all guilt and shame. However, I encourage patients to sit with those feelings. To identify where those feelings stem from. Guilt and shame are not always the enemy. Perhaps the patient feels guilty because they took advantage of someone sexually, or maybe they feel shame because they did not hold to their sexual values. In each of these instances, guilt and shame are warranted and should be used to help the patient grow in a way that respects who they want to be as sexual beings. The problem is not when we experience guilt and shame based on our convictions but when we experience guilt and shame based upon the convictions that others place on us.

Step Two – Uncover

The next step is to **uncover** any underlying issues that are connected with the patient's faith. As mentioned above, when it comes to guilt and shame, it may not be directly tied to the patient's religious beliefs or any specific religious teachings; however, that does not mean there cannot be some connection. For example, if an Orthodox Jewish patient presented with complaints of early ejaculation, it would be easy to speculate that his shame comes from finishing too quickly. Perhaps one could imagine this as a source of embarrassment or that the patient finds it emasculating. Yet, by understanding his religious beliefs, the clinician can uncover issues that are connected to his faith which could be the source of the guilt and shame. In this instance, understanding the religious prohibition against ejaculating outside of the vagina could be a contributing factor. Or, understanding that part of the marital obligations of the husband to his wife is to provide her with sexual satisfaction. Both of these could be contributors to the guilt and shame the patient feels.

Step Three – Recognize

Next, one should strive to **recognize** ethical concerns, dilemmas, and personal biases related to religion, specifically that of the patient's religious beliefs. This step can be extremely tricky as there are a lot of multi-faceted variables to consider. Let us consider a patient who perhaps has multiple wives. There are ethical concerns and dilemmas that arise from this. For example, what are the legalities of polygamy in the area in which you practice? Issues concerning therapist bias also arise from this. How do you, as a therapist, feel about polygamy? In my experience, through talks I have given to both American and European audiences, even those who accept and support polyamory have negative reactions when I discuss polygamy.

In addition to addressing the specific issues brought up in therapy, clinicians must also be mindful of their potential biases against their patients' autonomy, particularly in cases where religion is a contributing factor to the patient's decision-making process. This is particularly evident when working with religious patients who are grappling with their sexual orientation and express a desire to live as heterosexual despite being gay. For clinicians who identify as part of the LGBTQ+ community, or advocate for this community, this can be a difficult and emotional situation to navigate.

There is also the issue of countertransference that a therapist must consider when working with religious patients. This refers to the therapist's unconscious emotional reaction or response to the patient that is based on the therapist's own experiences, beliefs, and values. In the context of working with religious patients, countertransference can be manifested in two different ways. The first way is when the clinician holds no particular religious tradition or may even reject religion altogether and encounters a patient who is religious, as discussed in Chapter 1. The second way is when a clinician holds to a particular religious tradition that opposes the religious tradition of the patient. This form of countertransference can also manifest when the clinician and the patient are of the same faith tradition but belong to different sects or denominations. In either of these situations, there is a clash of worldviews and belief systems that can be a cause for serious ethical concerns that can impede progress in therapy. Therefore, as a helping professional, it is crucial to remain vigilant and acknowledge any ethical concerns, dilemmas, potential biases, or limitations that may arise during therapy sessions.

Step Four – Develop

The final step is to **develop** a path for the patient to reach congruency between their religious beliefs and their sexual behavior. What congruency looks like for each patient is different and should be based upon the patient's individual goals and not the goals, hopes, and desires of the clinician. For example, when dealing with a religious patient who is struggling with their sexual orientation, as "sex-positive" clinicians, we may feel congruency is the patient just accepting and embodying that orientation and finding a religious community that will accept them or leaving their religious tradition altogether. However, that may not be what the patient wants. Perhaps they like their religious community. Perhaps they like their faith tradition and believe in it strongly. The goal is to help the patient find congruency in the way that they choose to live their life.

There are three important elements that should be included when helping the patient reach congruency, (a) psychosexual education, (b) incorporating the patient's faith tradition in the therapeutic process, and (3) finding creative solutions.

As previously discussed, psychosexual education falls under the limited information part of the PLISSIT model. It is not uncommon for religious patients to need psychosexual education in understanding both their and their partner's sexual and reproductive anatomy, sex and sexuality in general, and in developing sexual communication skills. It has been my experience that psychosexual education with religious patients should be conducted in the early sessions of treatment so that the patient will be better equipped to discuss issues within therapy.

The second important element that should be incorporated is the patient's faith tradition. There have been some researchers and authors who have suggested that biblical teachings and theological concepts should be reframed in a more sex-positive light (Hung & Jung, 2009; Dale & Keller, 2019). However, I reject this notion due to its limited application and efficacy. Such models only work when the patient is not from a strongly conservative faith background and is not actively involved in their religious community.

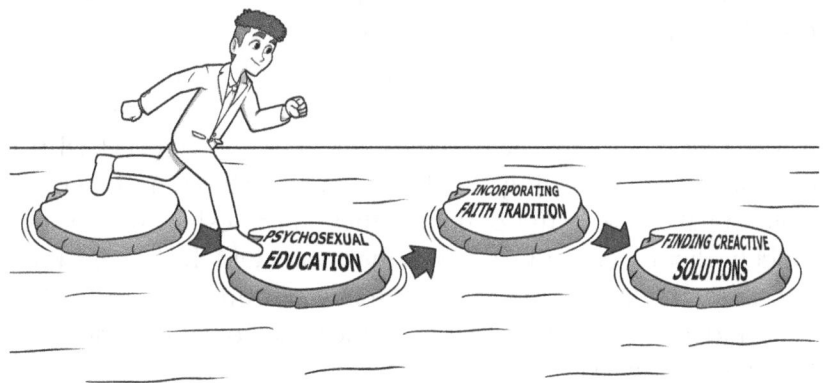

PATH TO CONGRUENCY

FIGURE 3.3 The path to congruency.

For individuals coming from conservative religious communities, alternative interpretations of sacred texts may be perceived as heretical and therefore rejected outright. This may also result in a lack of trust or confidence in the therapist's ability to understand and address their religiously informed concerns. However, despite these potential barriers, it is still possible for clinicians to have productive discussions with patients about their understanding of sacred texts.

Instead of reframing sacred texts in a sex-positive lens, in an attempt at "Sex Therapists Eisegesis," it can be much more helpful to ensure that the patient is reading the passages in context. The term "in context" can seem very vague, of course, so it becomes important to specify what is meant. Reading the Bible in context means reading and interpreting the meaning of biblical passages based on the historical, cultural, and literary context in which they were written. This involves understanding the original language and considering the literary genre of the text, as well as the historical and cultural background in which it was written. It also involves examining the text in relation to other passages in the Bible.

First, it is important that the text is being read in the context of the chapter and book in which it is found. An example would be a Pentecostal Holiness patient I worked with, who continued to quote a text from the Hebrew Bible/Old Testament which says, "Consecrate yourselves therefore, and be holy, for I am holy" (English Standard Version Bible, 2018, Leviticus 11:44). They frequently used this verse to solidify their position that they must refrain from all sexual behaviors until marriage. However, to me, it was a bit confusing because the context of the verse is kashrut, or teachings concerning what foods are and are not permissible to eat. I asked the patient if they kept kosher, which they quickly dismissed and said that that was "Old Testament law" and they are "not living under the law but under grace." They were indeed shocked when I explained the context of the verse they kept quoting.

A verse's meaning can also be taken out of context when it is not understood within the whole of the sacred canon. For example, certain biblical authors already assume that you read and are familiar with earlier writings (i.e., the prophets have assumed that the reader has read the Torah). Therefore their writings must be understood within the context the author intended, recognizing the greater scope of sacred text. Many Christian patients will understand this principle by mentioning how the New Testament authors often quote from the Old Testament.[1] Thus we see the greater context is essential in understanding what the author meant when referencing it.

With any ancient texts, including the Bible and the Quran, it is necessary to recognize the role of **hermeneutics**. Within the discipline of hermeneutics, one examines the interpretation of a text. This could be in light of understanding the nuances of the original language in which the document was written, as well as understanding the cultural and social climate in which the original author lived while writing to the original audience (Brown, 2021). Comparisons can also be made between texts, such as between the Quran and the Bible (Galadari, 2018).

As an example of how this works, my doctoral dissertation in biblical studies at the University of Mainz was in the Hebrew Bible, biblical archaeology, and psychological exegesis. The subject involved analyzing the way sex, sexuality, and gender were thought of in the Ancient Near East. In order to accomplish this, I examined archaeological remains, paying close attention to the iconographic depictions of sexual interaction, which gave insight into the way that the ancient craftsperson thought about sex. Additionally, I explored biblical and extrabiblical[2] sources, the latter of which acted as a commentary for the biblical text.

What my research led to was the discovery of *why* certain prohibitions concerning sex are included in the biblical texts. The purpose of such prohibitions was then explored through cross-textual examination, providing further evidence to support my theories. Such understanding can be exceptionally helpful in clinical practice because it allows us to share information with the patient that does not contradict what the biblical texts say but contradicts the way in which the biblical texts were previously understood. This is a position that most fundamental and conservative religious individuals would understand and accept.

The final element is providing creative solutions that the patient can incorporate without contradicting their religious convictions. Though it has been mentioned several times that some therapists encourage their patients to abandon religious practice, it must be stated that such a solution is a lazy option. This suggestion does not require that the clinician do any creative thinking or display any problem-solving abilities. It is much easier to tell a female Muslim patient, "leave your faith so that you can use this vibrator and finally have an orgasm," than to find a solution that works within the framework of her faith tradition. Likewise, it is much easier to tell an Orthodox Jewish man to leave his faith tradition so that he can masturbate to overcome early ejaculation than to find a creative solution that works within the framework of his faith tradition.

Working with religious patients requires additional attention and consideration that may not be necessary for other patients. However, the process of developing critical thinking, thoughtful analysis, and problem-solving skills for working with religious patients can lead to better, more insightful, and compassionate clinicians. These are valuable skills that can be utilized when working with patients from all cultural and religious backgrounds. By learning to approach religious patients with an open mind, therapists can develop a deeper understanding of their patient's beliefs and values, as well as the ways in which these beliefs may impact their mental health and well-being. This approach allows therapists to work collaboratively with their patients to identify areas of concern and develop effective treatment plans that are consistent with the patient's religious and cultural beliefs. Ultimately, this leads to better outcomes and greater patient satisfaction.

Incorporating these three steps is not an easy task, but it is essential for helping patients achieve a state of congruency. Congruency, in this context, refers to a sense of harmony and alignment between one's inner experiences and outer behaviors. However, it is important to note that the therapist should not impose their own definition of congruency onto the patient but rather help the patient discover their own sense of congruency. This is achieved by fostering an environment of acceptance and self-actualization, where the patient feels empowered to make their own decisions regarding their sexuality, sexual orientation, and gender identity within their religious context. It takes time and practice to create a therapeutic environment that promotes these elements, but the result is a positive and empowering therapeutic relationship.

Conclusion

The presented protocol in this chapter offers a valuable framework for therapists to effectively engage with religious individuals and couples. However, it is important to recognize that the application of the protocol will vary depending on the specific beliefs and practices of each patient's faith tradition, which will be further explored in subsequent chapters of this book. Therapists must strive to develop a foundational understanding of the patient's religious background, as discussed in Chapter 2, and continue to explore the dynamic relationship between their religious observance and sexual beliefs. This ongoing exploration is essential for tailoring treatment approaches and ensuring a more comprehensive understanding of the patient's experiences.

While having a protocol specifically designed for working with religious patients can be empowering for clinicians, it is important to acknowledge the limited availability of models in this area until recent times. Traditional approaches, such as reframing biblical texts from a sex-positive or feminist perspective, may not resonate with patients from fundamentalist and conservative faith traditions who adhere strictly to teachings within their denomination. Instead, it is recommended to approach sacred texts by examining them within their historical, cultural, and socio-economic contexts. This approach allows for more meaningful engagement with the patient and fosters open dialogue about their concerns related to sex, sexuality, and gender, which are influenced by their religious beliefs. By taking this approach, therapists can overcome resistance and create a safe space for those they work with to explore and reconcile their religious and sexual identities.

Notes

1 Though time and space does not allow for it here, an entire discussion can be had on if the New Testament authors correctly quote the Hebrew Bible/Old Testament text. While it is only advised that clinicians with strong command of biblical and other sacred texts undertake such discussions with patients, it should still only be used as a last result since it could cause the patient to have a crisis of faith if they determine that their sacred text is incorrect and misleading.
2 The term "extrabiblical" refers to sources that are outside of the Bible.

References

Annon, J. S. (1976). The PLISSIT model: A proposed conceptual scheme for the behavioral treatment of sexual problems. *Journal of Sex Education and Therapy, 2*(1), 1–15.

Brown, J. K. (2021). *Scripture as Communication: Introducing Biblical Hermeneutics*. Baker Publishing Group.

Currid, J. D., & Chapman, D. W. (Eds.). (2018). *ESV Archaeology Study Bible*. Crossway Books.

Dale, B., & Keller, R. (2019). *Advancing Sexual Health for the Christian Client: Data and Dogma*. Taylor & Francis.

Dubinskaya, A., Horwitz, R., Scott, V., Anger, J., & Eilber, K. (2023). It is time for doctors to Rx vibrators? A systematic review of pelvic floor outcomes. *Sexual Medicine Reviews, 11*(1), 15–22. DOI: 10.1093/sxmrev/qeac008

Galadari, A. (2018). *Qur'anic Hermeneutics: Between Science, History, and the Bible*. Bloomsbury Publishing.

Hunt, M. E., & Jung, P. B. (2009). "Good sex" and religion: A feminist overview. *Journal of Sex Research, 46*(2/3), 156–167. DOI: 10.1080/00224490902747685

Rash, J. K., Seaborne, L. A., Peterson, M., Kushner, D. M., & Sobecki, J. N. (2023). Patient reported improvement in sexual health outcomes following care in a sexual health clinic for women with cancer. *Supportive Care in Cancer, 31*(3). DOI: 10.1007/s00520-023-07635-4

PART II

What Every Therapist Should Know about Religion

Overview

To engage effectively with religious patients, clinicians should possess a foundational understanding of the specific faith tradition to which their patients belong. In this section, comprehensive insight into each of the Abrahamic faiths is provided, delving into pivotal sex-related principles intertwined with their sacred texts.

Learning Objectives

♦ Explain the core differences between Judaism, Christianity, and Islam.
♦ List the three essential sacred texts in Judaism, Christianity, and Islam.
♦ Discuss the significance of cultural variations and individual beliefs within each faith tradition.
♦ Evaluate the potential impact of religious beliefs on an individual's perception of their own sexuality and their ability to engage in a therapeutic process effectively.

DOI: 10.4324/9781003242017-6

4

Judaism and Sex

Introduction

Jews are commonly referred to as "the people of the book." This is a reference to the Jewish people's connection with the Bible, more specifically, the Hebrew Bible – also known as the Torah or the Tanakh. While the Torah is the name given to the first five books of the Hebrew Bible (Genesis, Exodus, Leviticus, Numbers, and Deuteronomy), it is sometimes used in more traditional communities to mean all biblical texts.

The Tanakh, on the other hand, always refers to the entirety of the Hebrew Bible. The word Tanakh acts as an acronym for *Torah*, *Nevi'im*, and *Ketuvim*, the three divisions of the Hebrew Bible. These are the same books found within the first three-fourths of the Christian Bible, known as the Old Testament, though the order in which the individual books appear is different. While there are similarities between the two canons, when working with Jewish patients, therapists should refrain from using the term "Old Testament" when referring to the Hebrew Bible. The term is often seen as offensive as it carries theological implications (Brettler, 2007, 7–8).

Jewish tradition teaches that when God gave the Torah to Moses and the Children of Israel on Mount Sinai, two Torahs, or Torot, were given – one written, as preserved in the biblical text, and the other verbally, known as the Oral Torah. The Oral Torah provides an explanation and further detail not found within the

DOI: 10.4324/9781003242017-7

biblical text. For example, Exodus 20:8 instructs to, "Remember the Sabbath day, to keep it holy." But what does that mean? How do you remember the Sabbath day? How do you keep it holy? The oral Torah provides that instruction.

Another example is Deuteronomy 12:21, which says, "then you may kill any of your herd of your flock, which the Lord has given you, *as I have commanded you*, and you may eat within your towns whenever you desire." While the text states that instructions have been given on how to slaughter an animal, the written Torah does not provide those details. However, the oral Torah does (Donin, 2019, 26). Thus, the oral Torah has become an important reference for observant Jews to better understand the written texts.

Originally, the oral Torah was passed down from generation to generation. However, ancient Rabbis eventually decided that it needed to be written down for fear of the traditions being lost. These laws and traditions were compiled and edited in written format between the third and sixth centuries in a volume known as the Talmud. In actuality, the Talmud is a collection of two books known as the Mishnah and the Gemara. The Mishnah is the oral Torah in written form and the Gemara is a rabbinical commentary on the former (Steinsaltz, 2006, 114–117). These collections of texts make up the foundation for all of Jewish thought and teaching.

Judaism is divided into several sects; however, these sects, as we know them today, did not emerge until the nineteenth century. These three major sects of Judaism are known as Orthodox, Conservative, and Reform. Within each of these movements, there are also subsects, which range in levels of observance to Jewish tradition and Jewish law – known as *halakhah*. Therefore the term "orthodox" does not represent a monolithic group (Friendman, 2019). It may be helpful to imagine a spectrum ranging from completely secular to extremely religious and observant. Those who are more observant in their practice of Judaism are often referred to as being frum. The word *frum* is Yiddish and is derived from the German word "froom," which means religious or pious.

It is necessary when working with a Jewish patient to inquire about their level of observance. The Orthodox will be the more religiously observant, whereas the Reform will be much less so. Do not be surprised to find great disparity ranging from those who go to the synagogue twice a year for the high holidays to those who may even go multiple times a day for prayer. The more observant the patient typically indicates how great of a role the Torah and Talmud take on in their daily lives. As such, these texts will inform the way that the Jews think about sex, sexuality, and gender.

The Purpose of Sex within Judaism

Judaism views sexual urges as natural (Steinsaltz, 2006, 180). It is a basic need and desire and is considered just like any other need or desire that a person may have. As such, it is not seen as inherently wrong, evil, or sinful. The purpose of sex within Judaism is twofold: (1) procreation and (2) pleasure. The emphasis on procreation comes from the first *mitzvah*, or commandment, found within the Hebrew Bible.

> And God blessed them, and God said to them, Be fruitful, and multiply, replenish the earth, and subdue it: and have dominion over the fish of the sea, and over the birds of the air, and over every living thing that moves on the earth.
>
> Genesis 1:28 (*Koren Tanakh*)

Considering the strong emphasis that Judaism places on the family, it is perhaps without much surprise that procreation is considered important. Most religiously observant Jews will strive to have at least two children – one of each sex. It would also not be uncommon for them to have additional children. Judaism also emphasizes the pleasure aspect of sex. The Torah, Talmud, and even the wedding contract, known as the *ketubah,* all speak about pleasure during sexual interactions between couples. More specifically, a focus is placed on the woman's sexual pleasure and fulfillment, beginning with the biblical texts:

> If he take another wife for himself; her food, her clothing, and her sexual rights, he shall not deminish.
>
> Exodus 21:10

The three elements mentioned in Exodus 21:10 are included in the *ketubah*, providing a guarantee of sexual enjoyment for the woman. Recognizing how men and women respond differently and have different needs sexually, the Talmud encourages foreplay for female arousal (Nedarim 20a) and men are even instructed to focus on their partner's pleasures so that they orgasm first (Niddah 31a–b). The idea of sexual pleasure is a holy pursuit. Maimonides, one of the greatest Jewish commentators of all time, suggested in *Mishneh Torah* (Shabbat 30:14) that sexual relations were a part of Sabbath pleasure (Steinsaltz, 2017).

Jewish Views on Sex Before Marriage

While it is common to hear that sex before marriage is prohibited within Judaism, the concept of sex before marriage is actually a modern concept, and as such, it is not found in neither the Torah nor the Talmud. Ancient marriages did not include the pomp and circumstance that accompany the tradition today. The idea of wedding parties and ceremonial events is a more modernized conceptualization of the union between partners. The Talmud speaks of marriage as an acquisition, emphasizing the legality of the exchange: "She is acquired through money, through a document, and through sexual intercourse" (Kiddushin 2a:1).

It should be noted that while such terminology may be shocking to our modern ideas about relationships, contrary to the notion that such laws are oppressive toward women, these laws are established for the protection of those women existing in a time when living conditions were harsh and survival was difficult. Within ancient Jewish society, a woman still had autonomy over her sexuality and within her relationship. A woman could not be forced to have sex (Eruvin 100b:14) and women had the ability to acquire a divorce, known as a *get*, from their husband on their own (Kiddushin 2a:2).

Nevertheless, *halachically* speaking, two people who engage in sexual intercourse before they are married, whether or not they had a modern ceremony, would require a *get* before marrying another partner. Another element to consider when speaking of sexual relations before marriage is that of the ritual bath known as a *mikveh*. The *mikveh* is an important part of most Orthodox women's lives, beginning shortly before their wedding day. It is required of a Jewish woman to immerse in the waters of the *mikveh* before they engage in sexual activity, both for the first time and following periods of menstruation (which will be discussed later). Once she is immersed in the water, she is then prepared for sexual interactions with her partner. Some may believe that it is the failure to engage in this ritual bathing that actually prohibits the sexual union between two people who are not married and conclude that sexual relations would be permissible if the female partner did immerse in the *mikveh*.

In more traditionally observant communities, there may be restrictions on unmarried men and women being alone together. This separation of the sexes is intended to eliminate the possibility that the two may engage in sexual behavior or even handholding in some cases. However, this attitude should not be taken as the norm. Various communities have adopted a wide range of what is deemed as appropriate, acceptable, or allowable behavior. As Cohn-Sherbook et al. (2013, 16) mention, "Rather than being kept separate, it is universally accepted – except among the strictly Orthodox – that young Jewish men and women will go out together and engage in various degrees of sexual activity before marriage." Thus, it would not be uncommon, even among Orthodox couples, to learn that the couple engaged in some form of physical intimacy before marriage.

Jewish Views on Sex Within Marriage

Marriage is a central component of Jewish life. In fact, it is considered the nucleus of all life (Steinsaltz, 2006, 181). This is a foundational principle held by both Orthodox and non-Orthodox Jewish communities. Within the boundaries of the marital relationship, Judaism teaches that sex should be enjoyed regularly for the pleasure of both bride and groom (Cohn-Sherbok et al., 2013, 3). However, it is the groom who assumes responsibility for his bride's sexual satisfaction as outlined in the *ketubah* (Lau, 2010, 371). This level of responsibility can sometimes add extra stress and anxiety to the male partner, especially when they lack sexual experience.

Generally speaking, it can be perceived that women have more autonomy over sexual interactions than their male counterparts. For example, a woman can deny her husband sex, although a husband is forbidden from denying his wife sexual satisfaction (Donin, 2019, 124). Women also have the option of using sex toys to enhance pleasure. These products can be used in solo or partnered sex, though preference is usually given to partnered sex.

The restriction from refusing sexual satisfaction to the woman extends beyond her capabilities to procreate – once again, demonstrating the important role pleasure has in the Jewish view of sex. Even if a woman has reached menopause, she is still entitled to sexual satisfaction from her partner (David & Weitzman, 2015). These very requirements emphasizing female sexual satisfaction benefit both husband and wife and help create connection and opportunities for bonding which will strengthen the longevity of the marriage.

When working with Orthodox Jewish couples on issues related to sexuality, it is necessary to be mindful of *Taharat HaMishpacha*, or family purity laws. These laws dictate that husband and wife must separate while she is menstruating and are based on the Torah:

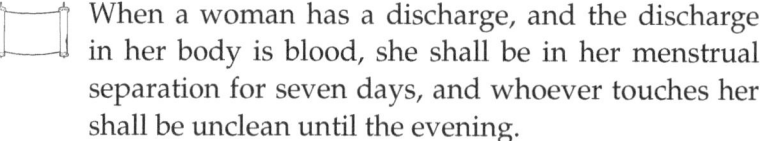 When a woman has a discharge, and the discharge in her body is blood, she shall be in her menstrual separation for seven days, and whoever touches her shall be unclean until the evening.

Leviticus 15:19

During this time, couples will refrain from all forms of physical intimacy, including touching and often sleeping in the same bed. This period of separation will generally last somewhere between twelve to fourteen days, from the beginning of menstruation until the woman immerses in the ritual bath, *mikveh*. The period of time is known as **niddah**, it is used to describe the woman who is menstruating or who has finished menstruating but has yet to immerse in the *mikveh*. The term *niddah* is used synonymously with *Taharat HaMishpacha*.

For a sex therapist, hearing concepts of purity and cleanliness related to a normal bodily function, such as menstruation, can seem shocking or even upsetting. However, I have found that the notion many people living in Western society have of purity and uncleanness is informed by an unrelated religious context. The context here is ritual purity. The classification of unclean does not equate to sin, morality, or value. Menstruation was not seen as something that is evil or bad (Loader, 2013, 76). It is a normal facet of life and when it transpires, a person needs to know what to do and how to respond.

The period of *niddah* is simply a time for a woman to separate from her partner so that she can focus her physical, emotional, and spiritual needs while at the same time being able to reset the sexual desire within the relationship. There are a few ways that could help non-Jewish therapists understand this concept, as there are similarities to modern sex therapy concepts. First, *niddah* is a time to focus on the emotional feelings and/or physical conditions of the woman (Donin, 2019, 125). Second, both partners are freed from the psychological burden and/or guilt that one partner may feel when rejecting the other partner's sexual advances. It also eliminates the feelings of rejection that the other partner often experiences since they recognize the rejection is based on religious conviction and is not a rejection of them personally (Donin, 2019, 126).

Finally, it has been stated that the *niddah* period has been shown to increase sexual desire and relational health within the partnership (Lau, 2010, 380). This period of sexual separation helps to element sexual boredom and routine within the marriage over periods of time (Donin, 2019, 126). It can also help to facilitate a deeper appreciation of the time they have to connect physically and not take it for granted. I would suggest this is also a period of time where a couple can focus on their emotional connection, something that is often overlooked. As sex therapists, we are often so focused on the essentiality of sex that we can easily overemphasize the need for sexual connection over other forms of connectedness. *Niddah* allows Jewish couples to focus on strengthening their connection in areas that extend beyond physical intimacy.

Jewish Views of Sex Outside of Marriage

It may be surprising to discover that the Torah actually permits polygamy, and additionally, the Talmud assumes that a man can have several wives (Steinsaltz, 2006, 127).[1] Nevertheless, polygamy is not something normally observed in modern Judaism.[2] This is due a *herem* (or ban) placed on polygamy by Rabbenu Gershom ben Judah of Mainz in the Middle Ages (Steinsaltz, 2006, 172). Therefore, it is rather uncommon to find modern Jewish families with multiple partners.

Since marriage within Judaism is exceptionally sacred, sexual encounters outside of the framework of marriage are viewed as "undermining this fundamental feature of Jewish life" (Cohn-Sherbok et al., 2013, 15). As such, polyamory is viewed negatively (Keshet-Orr & Collings, 2019, 12). Even if both partners consent, polyamory would be considered a form of infidelity despite any negotiations that the couple may have to the contrary.

The boundary against infidelity is clearly outlined within the biblical text:

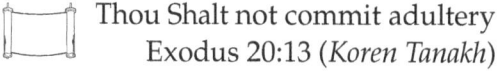 Thou Shalt not commit adultery
Exodus 20:13 (*Koren Tanakh*)

Such clear statements do not risk the possibility of falling victim to misinterpretation. No mental gymnastics are required to understand that infidelity is prohibited. The biblical law also requires punishment for acts of adultery:

> And the man that commits adultery with another man's wife, that commits adultery with his neighbour's wife, the adulterer and the adulteress shall surely be put to death.
>
> Leviticus 20:10 (*Koren Tanakh*)

While discussion about capital punishment for adultery may be troubling for most readers, it is primarily due to a lack of understanding of Jewish law, even among non-practicing Jews. In order for such punishment to actually be given, there are significant qualifications which have to be met. The Talmud details very specific requirements related to having witnesses, who the witnesses can and can not be, the responsibility of the witnesses, avoidance of hearsay, and the obligation to verbally warn the person committing the prohibited act. The very complex requirements to even reach a verdict of the death penalty are almost impossible. In fact, due to the stringencies, the Mishnah labels a religious court that executes one person within seventy years as destructive (Makkot 1:10).

Why, then, would such strong language be used in the biblical text? The purpose of such language is to emphasize the seriousness of the person's behavior and the effect their behavior has on others. It is not uncommon to hear those who were victims of an extramarital affair use vivid language such as, "It felt like my heart was ripped out of me," or "I felt like I died," to describe the way they felt when learning of their partner's infidelity. When weighing the importance that Judaism places on the family unit, it is easy to recognize the severity of damaging that union both temporally and spiritually.

Jewish Views of Other Sexual Behaviors

While the Torah does permit most sexual practices within the marital relationship, there are some boundaries that are placed for the purpose of elevating sexual activity to a place of holiness. It can be the case that these boundaries, or lack of understanding about these boundaries, can add to the patient's anxiety and misconceptions about sex. It is not uncommon to hear patients echo misconceptions about sex, such as it must be conducted with the lights off and in the missionary position (Keshet-Orr & Collings, 2019, 12). Yet, as has been discussed, most Jewish sources encourage a wide range of sexual behavior between partners. Still, there are some boundaries that clinicians should be aware of when working with the Orthodox Jewish population.

Masturbation

Male masturbation is discouraged within Orthodox Judaism. The **Shulchan Aruch**, or *Code of Jewish Law*, published in 1565, is the most widely accepted compilation of *halakhah* and is still in use today. The text describes the wasting of semen as a graver sin than any other mentioned in the Torah. Additionally, it says they are under a ban, referencing Isaiah 1:15, which states, "your hands are full of blood" (Cohn-Sherbok et al., 2013, 11).

While the *Shulchan Aruch* is mostly accepted and used by the more stringent forms of Orthodoxy in our present age, prohibitions against masturbation are still common. This phenomenon is primarily due to the biblical narrative of Onan and Tamar.

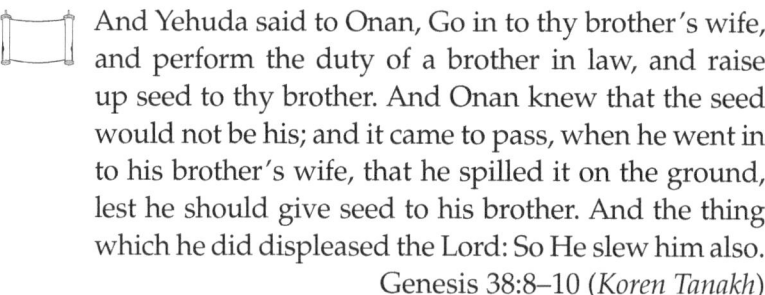

And Yehuda said to Onan, Go in to thy brother's wife, and perform the duty of a brother in law, and raise up seed to thy brother. And Onan knew that the seed would not be his; and it came to pass, when he went in to his brother's wife, that he spilled it on the ground, lest he should give seed to his brother. And the thing which he did displeased the Lord: So He slew him also.

Genesis 38:8–10 (*Koren Tanakh*)

The modern reader will most likely notice an unusual occurrence in this text — Onan was requested of his father to have intercourse with his sister-in-law. This was due to a cultural custom known as a ***levirate marriage***. The term *levirate* comes from the Latin *levir* meaning "husband's brother." A *levirate marriage* refers to the social obligation that the brother of a diseased person has toward his sibling's widow when there has not been an offspring. Such practices still take place in various parts of the world within clan-structured, agricultural-based societies.

In my forthcoming book, *Archaeology, The Bible, and Sex*, an argument is made concerning the wrongdoing recorded in this text. Was it the fact that Onan spilled his seed on the ground? Or was it that Onan refused to provide offspring for his brother, fulfilling his responsibility and ultimately taking advantage of Tamar by engaging in sexual relations with her under false pretenses? I conclude that the latter is the more validatable option in consideration of the context and clear reading of the text. Nevertheless, many Orthodox Jews hold to the boundary that ejaculation should only take place within the vagina. There is no textually recorded boundary concerning female masturbation.

Oral Sex

Oral sex is allowed within Judaism, as long as it falls within the previously mentioned boundaries. As such, fellatio is sometimes discouraged as it may cause a man to ejaculate outside of the vagina. Cunnilingus, on the other hand, is permitted and, in some recorded instances, even encouraged. For example, Maimonides, also known as the Rambam, wrote:

> A man may do whatever he wants with his wife. He may have intercourse with her at any time, and may kiss her on whatever limb of her body he wants. He may even engage in unnatural sex.
>
> Biah 21:10

Homosexuality

Keshet-Orr and Collings (2019, 12) state, "The Orthodox community is heteronominative in its attitudes to sex, with same-sex or multiple relationships seen only in critical or negative terms in Jewish law." However, the conversation about homosexuality is a bit more complex within Judaism than in other faith traditions. First, it is important to look at the foundational texts often referenced when speaking on the topic of homosexuality:

Do not have sexual intercourse with a man as with woman; it is an abhorrence.

Leviticus 18:22

If a man have sexual intercourse with a man like a woman, both of them have done an abhorrence; they shall die, their blood is upon them.

Leviticus 20:13

When considering the Jewish position on homosexuality held by the Orthodox community, there are two aspects that should be considered. The first consideration concerns what is actually prohibited according to the text. A clear reading of the text shows that there are no prohibitions recorded against homosexuality or homosexuals. The prohibitions mentioned in Leviticus are referencing a specific male-male sexual act (Drinkwater et al., 2009, 157). The second consideration concerns women and how the passages from Leviticus apply to female-female sexual acts. It is clear from these verses that there is no prohibition against female homosexuality (Rashkow, 2000, 31). In fact, the Rambam stated that there was no punishment for lesbianism in neither the biblical nor rabbinic law in his commentary to Mishnah Sanhedrin 7:4. Thus, most communities, even the most stringently observant, recognize that the boundaries described in Leviticus 18:22 and 20:13 are not specific to intrinsic attraction or identity but are in reference to one specific sexual act.

Gender Identity

Traditionally, Jewish thought tends to view the world in very binary ways (Robinson, 2016, 250). As such, it is perhaps not surprising that the issue of gender identity is not widely discussed within the Orthodox community (Keshet-Orr & Collings, 2019, 24). However, there are penalties for wearing the attire of the opposite sex, which is linked to marital laws and the prohibition of adultery (Cohn-Sherbok et al., 2013, 6). This boundary is based on the following teaching recorded in the Torah:

> A woman shall not wear a man's garment, nor shall a man put on a woman's cloak ...
>
> Deuteronomy 22:5

When dealing with the issue of gender identity, it is important to recognize an overriding principle in Judaism known as *pikuach nefesh*, a matter of *halakha* which states that the preservation of human life overrides all other religious restrictions, prohibitions, and obligations (Robinson, 2016, 100). This principle likewise applies to those dealing with gender dysmorphia. Under the principle of *pikuach nefesh*, a person may do what is necessary for their overall physical, mental, and emotional well-being.

At this point in time, all major branches of Judaism have, in some ways, encountered, and handled issues related to, or made statements concerning gender identity. For example, at the flagship Modern Orthodox institution, Yeshiva University, Dr. Joy Ladin is the David and Ruth Gottesman Chair in English at Sterns College for Women. Dr. Ladin is the first openly transgender person in such a position. Within the more progressive Jewish communities, both the Conservative and Reform movements have issued statements concerning the inclusion and acceptance of transgender persons in all aspects of Jewish life (Schreiber, 2016, 391).

In most circumstances, Jewish community leaders and rabbis are often seeking ways to help Jewish individuals be more involved in Jewish life inside of the community. This is an important element of the faith tradition. Even rabbis in the Talmudic times felt it was important to create space for all Jews to be included in religious and communal life regardless of various complications. In like manner, "many contemporary Jewish leaders and communities are committed to creating ways to include fully intersex, transsexual, and non-binary transgender Jews" (Robinson, 2016, 253–254).

Conclusion

Judaism is a diverse religion with a long and rich history. Unlike many other world religions that often avoid discussion about sex, sexuality, and gender, Judaism has never been shy in engaging in discourse around these topics. The Talmud records the tale of Rav Kahnah, who snuck into his teacher's house and hid under the bed in order to observe the way he interacted with his wife. He watched as they talked and laughed, as well as engaged in sexual relations. At some point, his teacher noticed Rav Kahnah hiding under the bed and chastised him, saying that his behavior was inappropriate and that he must leave. Rav Kahana responded, "This, too, is Torah, and I must learn" (Berakhot 62a:3).

The Jewish perspective on sex holds it in paramount importance within the human experience, viewing it as both ordinary and essential. Within this view, pleasure and intimacy are cherished components of the marital relationship, contributing to the development of the family and strengthening the bond between partners. The boundaries set by Judaism around sexual conduct are not intended for control or restriction but rather with the profound belief that these boundaries elevate what might be considered mundane, such as sexual interaction between partners, to a realm of holiness and beauty. As a helping professional, recognizing and respecting this perspective when working with Jewish individuals fosters a harmonious therapeutic alliance and enables the sensitive navigation of complex sexual and relational matters. Such an approach not only upholds their religious convictions but also contributes to their spiritual growth and enrichment.

Notes

1 The need for polygamy is outlined in my forthcoming book *Archaeology, the Bible, and Sex*. In short, in an agricultural society, polygamy was the norm, especially in the ancient world. It was a necessity to ensure the survival of the family. Many infants did not survive to adulthood and yet many children were needed to work the land and take care of other family businesses.

Additionally, in a time where there was no social security, children were expected to take care of their aging parents. Polygamy can still be observed today in many agricultural societies, including in the practice of a woman having more than one husband, known as *polyandry*, which is practiced in countries such as Tibet.

2 There are examples of polygamy being practiced by Jews from more predominantly Muslim nations. This was observed when Jews, from countries such as Azerbaijan, migrated back to their ancestral homeland of Israel in a process known as *aliyah*. In these cases it was not uncommon for them to have multiple wives, as was the custom from the area they migrated from. Thus, the nation of Israel had to make allowances to recognize their multiple spouses.

References

Brettler, M. Z. (2007). *How to Read the Jewish Bible*. Oxford University Press.

Cohn-Sherbok, D., Chryssides, G. D., & El Alami, D. S. (2013). *Love, Sex and Marriage: Insights from Judaism, Christianity and Islam*. SCM Press.

David, B. E., & Weitzman, G. A. (2015). Sexuality in advanced age in Jewish thought and law. *Journal of Sex & Marital Therapy, 41*(1), 39–48. DOI: 10.1080/0092623X.2013.811451

Donin, H. H. (2019). *To Be a Jew: A Guide to Jewish Observance in Contemporary Life*. Basic Books.

Drinkwater, G., Shneer, D., & Lesser, J. (Eds.). (2009). *Torah Queeries: Weekly Commentaries on the Hebrew Bible*. NYU Press.

Friedman, S. (2019). Assessing and treating sexual dysfunctions in orthodox Jewish couples: A summary of 41 consecutive cases. *Mental Health, Religion, & Culture, 22*(9), 930–942. DOI: 10.1080/13674676.2019.1688269

Keshet-Orr, J., & Collings, S. (2019). *In the Footsteps of the Fathers: Psychosexual Therapy with the Orthodox Jewish Community: An Overview from the Therapist's Chair*. Hakodesh Press.

Lau, Y. M. (2010). *Practical Judaism*. Modan Publishing House.

Loader, W. (2013). *Making Sense of Sex: Attitudes Towards Sexuality in Early Jewish and Christian Literature*. Eerdmans Publishing Company.

Rashkow, I. N. (2000). *Taboo or Not Taboo: Sexuality and Family in the Hebrew Bible*. Fortress Press.

Robinson, G. (2016). *Essential Judaism: A Complete Guide to Beliefs, Customs & Rituals*, updated edition. Atria Books.

Schreiber, G. (Ed.). (2016). *Transsexuality in Theology and Neuroscience*. De Gruyter.

Steinsaltz, A. (2006). *Essential Talmud*, thirtieth anniversary edition (C. Galai, Trans.). Basic Books.

Steinsaltz, A. (2017). *Rambam Mishne Torah Set*, 8 volumes. Toby Press.

5

Christianity and Sex

Introduction

For conservative Christians, the Bible plays a significant role in how they approach the world and those around them. The Christian Bible contains sixty-six books and is divided into two categories — the Old and New Testaments. The **Old Testament** is very similar in content, though not layout, to the Hebrew Bible. Within Protestant Christianity, the Old Testament contains thirty-nine books, whereas in Catholicism, it contains forty-six books, with the additional seven books coming from what is known as intertestamental period literature (Elwell & Yarbrough, 2022, 12–13). The New Testament contains twenty-seven books, four of which are known as the **Gospels** and tell of the life of Jesus, and thirteen (or possibly fourteen) were written by a very influential figure known as the Apostle Paul (Keown, 2021, 15).

In addition to the Old and New Testament, Mormons, those who are a part of the Latter Day Saints (LDS) movement, also hold that the Book of Mormon is inspired scripture (Givens, 2009, 70). The Book of Mormon is taught to be the writings of ancient prophets who lived between 600 BCE and 421 CE on the American continent. While there has been no archaeological or scientific evidence to support the claims made within the Book of Mormon concerning the peoples, places, and events recorded within, scholars within the movement strive to affirm the historicity of the texts (Gutjahr, 2012, 102–104).

DOI: 10.4324/9781003242017-8

For clarity, it should be mentioned that all other branches of Christianity reject the Book of Mormon (Davis, 2020, viii). In fact, due to the Latter-Day Saints' acceptance of the Book of Mormon, most fundamentalist and evangelical denominations label Mormonism as a cult and do not consider them to be a part of the Christian Church. Therapists, therefore, need to be mindful when working with Christians to avoid making comparisons between Mormonism and other fundamentalist denominations.

Within Protestant Christianity, there is a broad confessional sweep that ranges not only in doctrinal beliefs but in the way religious communities are set up and structured, as well as the amount of impact and influence the community has in the lives of parishioners. Even within a particular denomination, it is not unusual to recognize a high level of diversity in these areas. It is the responsibility of the therapist to discover their Christian patients' personal views on topics related to sex, sexuality, and gender and to notice how those views have been shaped by their particular religious community.

What is common within all of these denominations is the centrality of the biblical text. While more liberal denominations may not hold to the *inerrancy* and the *inspiration* of the Christian Bible, fundamentalist and conservative groups hold inerrancy and inspiration as core doctrines. Since American Christianity is largely comprised of these fundamentalist and conservative groups, it is most likely that presenting patients who identify as Christian have been influenced to some degree by the biblical text.

Often, Christianity is labeled as sex-negative. While there are some educators, counselors, and therapists who have tried to reframe the traditional Christian view of sex and sexuality by asserting that biblical texts have been taken out of context or should be viewed through a different lens, within the field of biblical scholarship their suggestions would quickly be discarded. Even more importantly, the conservative Christian seeking therapy would not accept what they would perceive as distortions of biblical truth. Such assertions could be interpreted as an attack on their religious beliefs and be the reason for them to abandon treatment altogether. Therefore, it is suggested that therapists avoid such tactics. However, this direction may work for individuals who have left their religious community but still self-identify as Christian.

Although Christianity has its roots in Judaism, the two religious traditions show distinct differences that go beyond their beliefs about the Messiah. Interestingly, one area where Judaism and Christianity diverge significantly is their perspectives on sexuality. Historically, Christians have sometimes resorted to using the more sex-positive views on sexuality held by Jews as a means to defame them (Drake, 2013). This revelation may come as unexpected to certain readers, underscoring the individuality of each tradition's stance on this matter. It also emphasizes the importance for clinicians to steer clear of generalizations when working with individuals from different religious backgrounds.

The Purpose of Sex Within Christianity

While today many mainstream Christian denominations recognize that sex is both for procreation and for pleasure, this has not historically been the case (Knust, 2006). Throughout history, Christianity has had a complex relationship with human sexuality, and its understanding of the purpose of sex has evolved over time.

In the early centuries of Christianity, there was a prevailing belief that sex was primarily for procreation within the bounds of marriage. This view was influenced by the writings of early Christian theologians, such as Augustine of Hippo, who emphasized the importance of sexual restraint and the control of desires (Augustine, 1996). According to this perspective, any sexual activity outside of marriage, for any other reason than procreation, was considered sinful and immoral. This was also true for masturbation. It is worth mentioning that Augustine, often considered one of the most significant early Church Fathers, famously converted to Christianity in 386 CE and was not only anti-Semitic in his theological writings but purposefully rejected Jewish teachings (Fredriksen, 2010).

It was not Augustine's anti-Semitic views that motivated his rejection of Jewish perspectives of sex and sexuality, but instead his adoption of Greek stoicism (Smith, 2011, 63). In fact, much of early Christian theology was the product of the incorporation of Greco-Roman philosophy and thought as outlined in Mark Edwards' *The Routledge Handbook of Early Christian Philosophy* (2021). This incorporation can be seen very early on in the Christian church's history and is referenced in the New Testament book of Acts and some of the epistles of Paul.

As Christian theology evolved and assimilated various cultural influences, a more refined understanding of the role of sex within the Christian tradition emerged. Naturally, this perspective varied across different denominational backgrounds and historical periods (Hessinger, 2022). While procreation continued to be regarded as significant, theologians increasingly recognized the value of sex in fostering intimacy and pleasure within a committed marital bond (Inserra, 2022).

Today, many Christian communities have embraced a more open and inclusive view of sexuality (Joyner et al., 2017). They recognize that sex can be an expression of love, intimacy, and mutual pleasure between partners, in addition to its procreative potential. This shift in perspective is often influenced by a more holistic interpretation of biblical teachings and an understanding of the importance of human flourishing and relational well-being.

However, it is essential to note that while many Christian communities have embraced these more inclusive views, the traditional positions on sex, which once held a systematic influence, still impact many modern believers, as it is intertwined in the theological traditions of their church and communities. The historical teachings on sexual morality continue to shape the beliefs and practices of some Christians, particularly those who adhere to more conservative or traditional interpretations of Scripture. It is important to highlight that the strong positions often labeled as "sex-negative" by therapists are not inherently problematic. The real issue lies in the way the community interprets, teaches, and enforces these beliefs.

Ultimately, the purpose of sex within Christianity is a subject of ongoing theological exploration and interpretation. Different

Christian denominations and individual believers may hold diverse views on the matter, but the underlying thread that unites them is the belief in the sacredness of human relationships, the significance of love, and the pursuit of a flourishing and ethical sexual expression within the boundaries of committed partnerships (Inserra, 2022). For most conservative Christians, the purpose of sex will be both for procreation and pleasure, the major difference will be what sexual acts they find permissible within the relationship.

Christian Views of Sex Before Marriage

Christianity places a very stringent boundary around sex before marriage. Traditional Christian teachings view sex before marriage as morally wrong and contrary to God's plan for human relationships (Cornelio & Claudio, 2022). This perspective is rooted in biblical passages that emphasize the sacredness of marriage and the importance of sexual purity.

One of the fundamental biblical teachings often cited in discussions on sex before marriage is found in the New Testament, in the writings of the Apostle Paul. In his letters, Paul urges believers to avoid sexual immorality and to maintain sexual purity. For example, in 1 Corinthians 6:18–20, Paul writes, "Flee from sexual immorality. All other sins a person commits are outside the body, but whoever sins sexually, sins against their own body. Do you not know that your bodies are temples of the Holy Spirit, who is in you, whom you have received from God?"

From this and other similar passages, many Christians understand that engaging in sexual activity before marriage is considered sinful because it violates the principle of sexual purity and the sacredness of the marital covenant (Inserra, 2022). It is believed that sexual intimacy is designed by God to be fully expressed within the committed and lifelong union of marriage, where it serves as a means of deepening the bond between husband and wife.

The reasons behind the Christian view of sex before marriage are rooted in a broader theological framework that emphasizes the importance of moral conduct, self-control, and the pursuit of holiness. Christians who hold to this view often argue that abstaining from premarital sex allows individuals to demonstrate discipline, respect for themselves and others, and obedience to God's commandments (Pedersen, 2014; Kansiewicz et al., 2022). However, while the boundaries around premarital sex seem to be shared among all conservative Christian denominations, it is not uncommon to find that young people engage in oral or anal sex in order to remain "virgins." This practice also took place among non-Jewish women in ancient times (Garroway, 2018, 35).

Christian Views on Sex Within Marriage

Christianity holds a rich and multifaceted view of sex within marriage, emphasizing its sacredness, purpose, and the importance of mutual love, respect, and intimacy between spouses. Within the context of a committed marital relationship, sex is seen as a gift from God that allows couples to express their love, strengthen their bond, and experience pleasure. The biblical teachings on marriage often highlight the significance of sexual intimacy as an integral part of the marital union. In the Old Testament, the Song of Solomon portrays the beauty and desire between a husband and wife, celebrating the physical and emotional aspects of their relationship. The New Testament also speaks to the importance of the sexual relationship within marriage, emphasizing the mutual responsibility and care between spouses.

The Apostle Paul, in his writings, provides guidance on the role of sex within marriage. In 1 Corinthians 7:3–5, he writes, "The husband should fulfill his marital duty to his wife, and likewise the wife to her husband. The wife does not have authority over her own body but yields it to her husband. In the same way, the husband does not have authority over his own body but yields it to his wife. Do not deprive each other except perhaps by mutual consent and for a time so that you may devote yourselves to prayer. Then come together again so that Satan will not tempt you because of your lack of self-control."

While this passage encourages married couples to engage in sexual activity with one another, how "sexual activity" is defined varies from community to community. Some will quote Hebrew 13:4, which states, "Let marriage be held in honor among all, and let the marriage bed be undefiled ..." and interpret the text to mean that any sexual act is allowed within the confines of marriage. Others, however, will argue that certain sexual acts (usually anal sex, labeled as sodomy) are not allowed. It is important to ask the patient what behaviors and practices they find acceptable and appropriate within the confines of the marital relationship.

Christian Views of Sex Outside of Marriage

As previously mentioned, Hebrews 13:4 is often interpreted to mean that all sexual acts within a marital relationship are allowed. The full verse states, "Let marriage be held in honor among all, and let the marriage bed be undefiled, for God will judge the sexually immoral and adulterous," and is often used to teach against adulterous relationships or any sexual encounter outside of the husband and wife. This would include polyamorous relationships, regardless of the consent of all partners.

This teaching holds an unequivocal foundation within the Christian doctrine. Notably, despite Christianity's disapproval of divorce, an exception is often given in the case of adultery (Patras & Usman, 2019). Such behavior is viewed as a moral failure or even viewed as some type of sexual disorder (Peters, 2022). Consequently, when infidelity occurs within a marital relationship, it triggers a complex interplay of profound emotional and psychological responses in both partners, encompassing a spectrum of intricate factors.

Christian Views of Other Sexual Behaviors

As most sexual health professionals will agree, the definition of sex extends far beyond that of intercourse (Hille et al., 2020).

Individuals engage in a wide range of sexual behaviors both with themselves and with their partners. As such, it is not surprising to discover that Christians often have a much more comprehensive perception of sex than some may assume due to their religious background. Additionally, it is worth noting that a person's acceptance or rejection of a certain behavior is not an indication of their sexual practices. As such, while a Christian patient may hold certain religiously informed sexual boundaries and yet not hold to those boundaries.

Masturbation

Within Christian communities, a diverse spectrum of perspectives prevails concerning the topic of masturbation, and a unanimous consensus remains elusive among adherents. The viewpoints on this matter exhibit a considerable breadth, encompassing staunch disapproval of the behavior on one end of the spectrum, to more lenient attitudes, mainly when it is considered as a substitute for premarital or homosexual intercourse. Notably, certain individuals within these communities assert that the practice may be indicative of addictive tendencies, warranting intervention and support from mental health professionals (Perry, 2019). Thus, it is vital to understand the perspective held by a Christian patient regarding masturbation when approaching the subject in a clinical setting.

Those who hold a more conservative stance often consider masturbation as a sinful act. They believe that the primary concern lies in the presence of lustful thoughts or fantasies that may accompany the act (Bernard, 1985, 252). These Christians draw upon passages such as Matthew 5:27–30, where Jesus addresses the issue of lust and emphasizes the importance of guarding one's thoughts and desires. According to this interpretation, indulging in sexual fantasies or using masturbation as a means of gratifying lustful desires is seen as contrary to God's commandments and a violation of the sacredness of human sexuality.

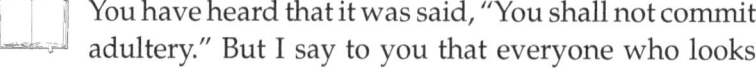 You have heard that it was said, "You shall not commit adultery." But I say to you that everyone who looks

> at a woman with lustful intent has already committed
> adultery with her in his heart. If your right eye causes
> you to sin, tear it out and throw it away. For it is better
> that you lose one of your members than that your
> whole body be thrown into hell. And if your right
> hand causes you to sin, cut it off and throw it away.
> For it is better that you lose one of your members than
> that your whole body go into hell.
>
> Matthew 5:27–30 (*English Standard Version*)

However, please note that not all Christian communities or individuals share this perspective. Some Christians take a more lenient or nuanced approach, acknowledging that sexual desires and impulses are a natural part of the human experience. They argue that masturbation, when done in moderation and without accompanying lustful thoughts, may be considered a morally acceptable means of finding release and relief from sexual tension.

In the absence of explicit biblical teachings directly addressing masturbation, different Christian traditions, and individuals draw upon broader principles and theological considerations to form their views. Some emphasize the importance of self-control, temperance, and the pursuit of purity in thought and action. They encourage individuals to examine their motives, attitudes, and the impact of their actions on themselves and their relationships with God and others.

Oral Sex

The views on oral sex, specifically fellatio (oral stimulation of the penis) and cunnilingus (oral stimulation of the female genitals), vary within different Christian communities. The biblical text does not specifically mention or discuss oral sex, though, not surprisingly, some scholars have tried to make such connections (Case, 2017). Early Christian teaching, however, held that oral sex "merited greater severity than anal sex" (Brundage, 1987, 167). Nevertheless, many Christians today hold the position that oral sex is acceptable within the marital relationship, using the Hebrews 13:4 argument.

Indeed, it is not uncommon to encounter Christian patients who hold divergent perspectives, particularly concerning the scope of acceptable sexual behaviors within the context of marital and pre-marital relationships. In certain Christian communities, a more permissive stance may be observed regarding the practice of oral sex, often viewed as an acceptable alternative to premarital intercourse. Conversely, there are those who maintain that such practices should be discouraged, even within the confines of a marital relationship. This underscores the significance of seeking clarification from the Christian patient regarding their specific beliefs and values in order to provide tailored therapeutic guidance. It is noteworthy to reiterate that the explicit discussion of this topic is notably absent within the canonical texts of the Old and New Testaments.

Homosexuality

Within certain fundamentalist and evangelical branches of Christianity, homosexuality is often viewed as morally unacceptable and condemned based on their interpretation of biblical teachings. This perspective stems from specific New Testament passages that address same-sex sexual activity:

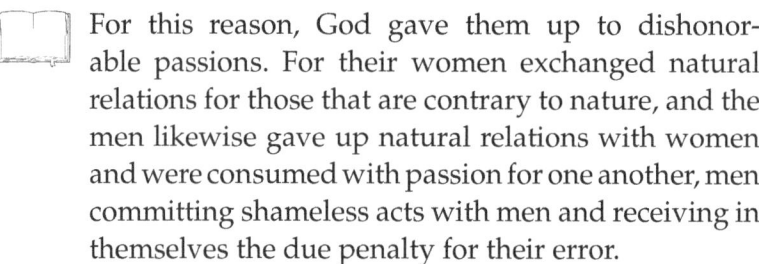

For this reason, God gave them up to dishonorable passions. For their women exchanged natural relations for those that are contrary to nature, and the men likewise gave up natural relations with women and were consumed with passion for one another, men committing shameless acts with men and receiving in themselves the due penalty for their error.

Romans 1:26–27 (*English Standard Version*)

Or do you not know that the unrighteous will not inherit the kingdom of God? Do not be deceived: neither the sexually immoral, nor idolaters, nor adulterers, nor men who practice homosexuality, nor thieves, nor the greedy, nor drunkards, nor revilers, nor swindlers will inherit the kingdom of God.

1 Corinthians 6:9–10 (*English Standard Version*)

> Understanding this, that the law is not laid down for the just but for the lawless and disobedient, for the ungodly and sinners, for the unholy and profane, for those who strike their fathers and mothers, for murderers, the sexually immoral, men who practice homosexuality, enslavers, liars, perjurers, and whatever else is contrary to sound doctrine.
>
> 1 Timothy 1:9–10 (*English Standard Version*)

The New Testament scriptures accentuate a significant divergence from the Old Testament regarding their treatment of homosexuality. In contrast to the Old Testament, the New Testament overtly condemns homosexuality as a whole, rather than specific sexual acts. Consequently, it is not uncommon to encounter individuals grappling with their sexual orientation who hail from conservative Christian backgrounds. Regrettably, a substantial portion of fundamentalist Christian denominations have shown limited receptiveness to the unique needs of LGBTQ individuals within their congregations, and certain denominations have been associated with practices such as conversion therapy (Clucas, 2017; Ogunbajo et al., 2022). Another prevalent response within the Christian community is to encourage members with same-sex attractions to embrace celibacy (Kansiewicz et al., 2022). Consequently, when confronted with community members exploring their sexual orientation, these matters are frequently either sidestepped or left unaddressed. It is pertinent to note that church disciplinary measures are typically invoked only when an individual openly acknowledges their same-sex attraction or is discovered engaging in same-sex behavior, albeit exceptions may exist.

Gender Identity

Traditional Christian teachings often stress a binary interpretation of gender, positing it as inherently dichotomous, rooted in the creation narrative found in the Book of Genesis. According to this narrative, it is believed that God fashioned humanity as "male and female" (Genesis 1:27). Consequently, this viewpoint traditionally aligns with a cisgender perspective, wherein an individual's gender identity aligns with the sex assigned at birth. Moreover, this binary framework significantly shapes expectations regarding gender presentation, particularly within more conservative and fundamentalist Christian denominations, where adherence to distinct modes of dress is often mandated, referencing guidelines found in the Old Testament:

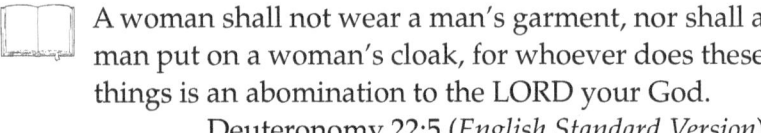 A woman shall not wear a man's garment, nor shall a man put on a woman's cloak, for whoever does these things is an abomination to the LORD your God.
Deuteronomy 22:5 (*English Standard Version*)

Based upon their interpretation of this text, actions as seemingly innocuous as women wearing pants can be perceived as deviating from the community's interpretation of biblical standards—often referred to as holiness standards (Bernard, 1985, 155–188). Although research at the intersection of religion and gender identity remains relatively limited, the existing body of evidence suggests a mixed impact of Christian communities on individuals with diverse expressions of sexuality (Kay et al., 2022). Notably, recent findings emphasize that gender-diverse Christians may experience harm stemming from the prevailing Christian stance of "love the sinner, but not the sin" (de Jong, 2020, 65). However, other studies point to the benefit of community support offered by the Christian church (Benson et al., 2018). This underscores the complex interplay between religious beliefs, gender identity, and the potential consequences for individuals within these communities.

Conclusion

Within Christian communities, perceptions of sex, sexuality, and gender exhibit significant variation. Liberal branches of Christianity tend to be more permissive, allowing for deviations from traditional doctrinal teachings. Conversely, conservative and fundamentalist sects maintain stricter standards of sexual behavior, rooted in their commitment to aligning with their interpretation of biblical texts.

Across these diverse Christian perspectives, specific common themes emerge regarding sexuality. Foundational principles such as love, respect, mutual consent, and the pursuit of holiness are consistently emphasized in the context of sexual relationships. Committed marital relationships, the cultivation of emotional and physical intimacy, and the recognition of the sacred nature of human sexuality are also central themes within many Christian viewpoints.

As Christians grapple with these complex issues, there is a growing recognition of the importance of fostering compassionate dialogue, engaging in profound theological reflection, and providing pastoral care to individuals and communities affected by differing views (Jacobson, 2023). This entails offering support and understanding to those facing challenges or conflicts related to their sexual orientation, gender identity, or adherence to traditional teachings. Ultimately, the aim of the clinician should be to help Christian patients to find congruency between their Christian faith and their sexual behavior.

In the ever-evolving landscape of human sexuality and gender identity, it is imperative to understand the intricate dynamics experienced by Christian individuals who grapple with these issues while maintaining their faith. It is vital to recognize that Christians do not adopt specific viewpoints on sex, sexuality, and gender to promote exclusion or reject others. Instead, their convictions are rooted in a profound belief that they are faithfully interpreting and aligning their lives with the teachings of the Bible. These individuals should be approached with empathy, respect, and a commitment to facilitating understanding within the intersection of their faith and the evolving societal norms regarding human sexuality and gender identity.

References

Augustine. (1996). *St. Augustine on Marriage and Sexuality* (E. A. Clark, Ed.). Catholic University of America Press.

Benson, K., Westerfield, E., & Van Eeden-Moorefield, B. (2018). Trans-gender people's reflections on identity, faith, and Christian faith communities in the U.S. *Sexual & Relationship Therapy*, *33*(4), 395–420. https://doi/10.1080/14681994.2018.1472375

Bernard, D. K. (1985). *Practical Holiness: A Second Look*. Word Aflame Press.

Brundage, J. A. (1987). *Law, Sex, and Christian Society in Medieval Europe*. University of Chicago Press.

Case, M. L. (2017). Cunning linguists: Oral sex in the song of songs. *Vetus Testamentum*, *67*(2), 171–186. DOI: 10.1163/15685330–12341277

Clucas, R. (2017). Sexual orientation change efforts, conservative christianity and resistance to sexual justice. *Social Sciences (Basel)*, *6*(2), 54. DOI: 10.3390/socsci602005

Cornelio, J., & Claudio, L. E. (2022). Waiting for "God's best": Love and sex in Evangelical Christianity in the Philippines. *Journal of Religion & Popular Culture*, *34*(2), 127–141. DOI: 10.31.38/jrpc.2021–0007

Davis, W. L. (2020). *Visions in a Seer Stone: Joseph Smith and the Making of the Book of Mormon*. University of North Carolina Press.

de Jong, D. H. (2020). *Conservative Christianity, Gender Identity, and Religious Liberty: A Primer and a Proposal*. Springer International Publishing.

Drake, S. (2013). *Slandering the Jew: Sexuality and Difference in Early Christian Texts*. University of Pennsylvania Press, Incorporated.

Edwards, M. (Ed.). (2021). *The Routledge Handbook of Early Christian Philosophy*. Routledge.

Elwell, W. A., & Yarbrough, R. W. (2022). *Encountering the New Testament: A Historical and Theological Survey* (W. A. Elwell, Ed.). Baker Publishing Group.

Fredriksen, P. (2010). *Augustine and the Jews: A Christian Defense of Jews and Judaism*. Yale University Press.

Garroway, K. H. (2018). *Growing Up in Ancient Israel: Children in Material Culture and Biblical Texts*. SBL Press.

Givens, T. (2009). *The Book of Mormon: A Very Short Introduction*. Oxford University Press, USA.

Gutjahr, P. C. (2012). *The Book of Mormon: A Biography*. Princeton University Press.

Hessinger, R. (2022). *Smitten: Sex, Gender, and the Contest for Souls in the Second Great Awakening*. Cornell University Press.

Hille, J. J., Simmons, M. K., & SANDERS, S. A. (2020). "sex" and the ace spectrum: Definitions of sex, behavioral histories, and future interest for individuals who identify as asexual, graysexual, or demisexual. *The Journal of Sex Research*, *57*(7), 813–8223. DOI: 10.1080/00224499.2019.1689378

Inserra, D. (2022). *Pure: Why the Bible's Plan for Sexuality Isn't Outdated, Irrelevant, Or Oppressive*. Moody Publishers.

Jacobson, C. (2023). *Abrahamic Faiths: Perspectives on Gender Identity and Sexuality*. Scholars' Press.

Joyner, A., Jordon, R. K., Johnson, J. M., & Barnhart, D. L. J. (2017). *Living Faithfully: Human Sexuality and The United Methodist Church*. Abingdon Press.

Kansiewicz, K. M., Zaporozhets, O., & Yarhouse, M. A. (2022). Sexual development, identity, and support for same-sex attracted celibate Christians. *Journal of Psychology and Christianity*, *41*(4), 253–264.

Kay, T. S., Wolff, J. R., Himes, H. L., & Alquijay, J. (2022). A retrospective qualitative analysis of christianity and its influence on gender identity development among transgender adults who were assigned female at birth. *Journal of Gay & Lesbian Mental Health*, *26*(3), 307–328. DOI: 10.1080/19359705.2021.1894297

Keown, M. J. (2021). *Discovering the New Testament: An Introduction to Its Background, Theology, and Themes (Volume II: the Pauline Letters)*. Lexham Press.

Knust, J. W. (2006). *Abandoned to Lust: Sexual Slander and Ancient Christianity*. Columbia University Press.

Ogunbajo, A., Oke, T., Okanlawon, K., Abubakari, G. M., & Oginni, O. (2022). Religiosity and conversion therapy is associated with psychosocial health problems among sexual minority men (SMM) in nigeria. *Journal of Religion and Health*, *61*(4), 3098–3128. DOI: 10.1007/s10943-021-01400-9

Patras, A. I., & Usman, A. (2019). Adultery, the ground for dissolution of christian marriage in pakistan: Intersectional constraint to Christian women in Pakistan. *Pakistan Perspectives*, *24*(2), 51.

Pedersen, W. (2014). Forbidden fruit? A longitudinal study of Christianity, Sex, and Marriage. *Journal of Sex Research*, *51*(5), 542–550. DOI: 10.1080/00224499.2012.753983

Perry, S. L. (2019). *Addicted to Lust: Pornography in the Lives of Conservative Protestants*. Oxford University Press.

Peters, P. E. (2022). Adultery as sexual disorder: An exegetical study of Matthew 5:27–30. *Hervormde Teologiese Studies*, *78*(4), 1–8. DOI: 10.4102/hts.v78i4.7577

Smith, J. W. (2011). *Christian Grace and Pagan Virtue: The Theological Foundation of Ambrose's Ethics*. Oxford University Press.

6

Islam and Sex

Introduction

In the early seventh century, Islam emerged on the Arabian peninsula in the city of Mecca, located in present-day Saudi Arabia (Ramadan, 2017, 1). The central religious text of Islam is the Quran. It is arranged in 114 surahs, or chapters, and is believed to be a direct revelation from God given to the prophet Muhammad by the archangel Gabriel. It should be very clear that observant Muslims do not simply believe that the Quran is inspired by God but that it is the literal word of God. The Quran is therefore considered co-eternal with God and, like God, has always existed (Sonn, 2011, 23). The oral revelations given to Muhammad did not begin until he was 40 years of age, in the year 610 CE, coinciding with the month of Ramadan. The revelations continued in a non-linear manner until his death 23 years later in 632 CE. It is believed that the prophet Muhammad was illiterate, however, God instructed him to share the teachings, which he did with those around him – resulting in the first converts to Islam, known as the Prophet's Companions. The Quran was not compiled into a written format until 633 CE, one year after the Prophet's death (Haleem, 2008, xi, xv–xvi.)

Within Islam, there is a special connection between the month of Ramadan and the Quran. Not only did Muhammad begin receiving revelations for the Quran during the month of Ramadan, but it is during Ramadan that observant Muslims

DOI: 10.4324/9781003242017-9

complete the recitation of the Quran during their *Tarawih* prayers and/or attempt to read the entire Quran. The term *tafsir* refers to the exegesis of the Quran. It is worth noting that the Muslim approach to *tafsir* is different from the approach taken by both Jews and Christians for interpreting their sacred texts (Peters, 2018, 94). Muslims typically rely on scholarly commentary to understand the Quran, in much the same way that religious Jews rely on commentary to understand the Torah. This is unlike most Christian denominations who focus more on direct translation of the texts. This is possibly due to the Christian premise that Jesus was his own revelation (Peters, 2018, 94).

As Sonn (2011, 23) notes, "Islam shares the history, basic beliefs, and values of Judaism and Christianity." Similar to Christianity, which believes that it is a continuation or fulfillment of Judaism, Muslims consider Islam as a successor of Judaism and Christianity. Islam has a very deep and abiding respect for Judaism and Christianity (Kaltner, 2016, 56). In fact, both Jews and Christians are referred to as *Ahl al-Kitab*, or "people of the book" in Islam (Rassool & Khan, 2020, 232). Muhammad, however, is considered to be *Rasūl Allah*, the final messenger sent from God to humanity (Ramadan, 2017, 5).

Since its inception, Islam has become an exceptionally diverse religion. Though it was founded on the Arabian peninsula, today, less than one-fifth of practicing Muslims live in an Arabic speaking nation (Kaltner, 2016, 9). Nevertheless, as Ramadan (2017, 99) explains, "Islam's unity arises from the fact that Muslims, be they Sunni, Shi'a, or Ibadi, or of whatever culture – Arab, African, Asian, or Western – or trend of thought – literalist, traditionalist, reformer, mystic – agree on the fundamental principles of their religion – the oneness of God, its scriptural sources, the creed. They also agree on its ritual practices and its essential obligations and prohibitions." In terms of creed, Islam can be summed up in five foundations of Islamic practices known as the Five Pillars of Islam (Blair & Bloom, 2002, 35).

The first of the five Pillars of Islam is known as the *shahāda*, and states, "there is no god [i.e., nothing worthy of worship] other than God, and the Prophet Muhammad is His messenger" (Ibrahim, 2022, 1). The second pillar, or *rukn*, is prayer, known as *salāt*. In order to keep this tenant of the faith, devout Muslims pray five times daily – including dawn, midday, sunset, dusk, and nighttime (Sonn, 2011, 40). The third *rukn* is *zakāt*, or charity, followed by *sawm*, fasting. The final *rukn* is *hajj*, or the obligation to make a pilgrimage to Mecca at least once in their lifetime, provided that they are physically and financially able to do so.

When it comes to the pillar of fasting, it is relevant to note that most Muslims fast during the month of Ramadan. This fast includes refraining from food and drink from sunrise to sunset each day of the month, and any behaviors or actions that are excessive in terms of their emotional reaction and impact on others. Additionally, Muslims abstain from sex during fasting hours, As Blair & Bloom (2022, 37) explain, "Abstinence during Ramadan brings Muslims greater awareness of God's presence and helps them acknowledge their gratitude for God's provision in their lives." This is exceptionally relevant and important as we begin to explore conceptions of sex within Islam.

The early revelations Muhammad received centered on topics such as monotheism, the principles of faith, the evils of adultery, and the afterlife. However, in 622 CE the Muslim community was forced to flee Mecca due to persecution and resettlement in Medina. From this time, the revelations began to deal with practical issues such as marriage and divorce (Cohn-Sherbok et al., 2013). While these revelations are recorded in the Quran, the Quran is not a collection of laws nor is it a body of legislation. For Sunni Muslims, the **Shari'a** (a practical set of guidelines for everyday Muslim life; shari'a translates as "path, road, or the way" and is to not be mistaken as Islamic law/fiqh) comes from the Quran and a collection of **hadith**, or narrations heard from the Prophet by his close companions, containing the words and deeds of the Prophet Muhammad. In the eighth and ninth centuries CE, these *ahadith* were divided into six authoritative collections, however, following the death of the Prophet, it became necessary for religious scholars to develop a set of principles for jurisprudence (Cohn-Sherbok et al., 2013, 34–35). Jurists are typically divided into four schools of thought named after the most prominent scholars – the Hanafi, Hanbali, Maliki, and Shafi'i. Two additional schools of thought also arose and continue to be prevalent today — are Salafis and Wahhabis. Both of which tend towards more literal and puritanical interpretations of the Quran and *hadith*. (Muhammad, 2017). Shi'a Muslims, on the other hand, accept only the words that can be traced back to the Prophet Muhammad and his immediate family, as well as a more limited range of jurisprudence for their basis for rulings.

Since jurisprudence on a topic depends not only on the division of Islam that one practices but also on the school of thought within that tradition, it is difficult to give a definitive guide to sex within Islam. However, it is possible to give a general overview solely based on Quranic texts and authenticated *hadiths*.

The Purpose of Sex within Islam

Islam teaches that sexual desire is natural and that sex should be pleasurable for both men and women. It is viewed as a time for bonding between partners and is elevated to a spiritual dimension. Of course, sex is also seen as a vehicle for procreation, something that is highly valued in Islam, since the faith places great value on the role and importance of the family. Thus, the sexual connection between partners, either for procreation or for pleasure, is seen as something that is both sacred and special.

As with all Abrahamic faith traditions, Islam places boundaries around certain aspects of sex, primarily who and when a person engages in sex. While specifics will be discussed in the sections below, there are some general prohibitions to be aware of. One such instance is the prohibition against having sex when menstruating or having sex with someone who is menstruating.

 And they ask you about menstruation. Say, "It is *harm*, so keep away from wives during menstruation. And do not approach them until they are pure. And when they have purified themselves, then come to them from where Allah has ordained for you. Indeed, Allah loves those who are constantly repentant and loves those who purify themselves."

Quran 2:222

Like in Judaism, Muslims are prohibited from having sex during menstruation. When a female is menstruating, she is considered to be in a state of impurity. This is not an indication that the woman is bad or evil and should be interpreted as such. It is simply a statement that she has arrived at a point where ritual purification is required. It is considered a normal and regular part of life. During the period of menstruation, she is to refrain from sexual intercourse, but other forms of sexual intimacy are not only encouraged but are demonstrated in detail within hadiths narrated by one of the Prophet's wives, Aisha. While such prohibitions may be unpopular among "sex-positive" social media influencers and sex educators, recent medical studies show that sex during menstruation could be connected with endometriosis, sexually transmitted diseases, an increase in menstrual blood, and unwanted pregnancy (Mazokopakis, 2020).

Sexual relations are also prohibited during the *hajj* or pilgrimage. This prohibition is in place so that the individual may focus on the spiritual development of the pilgrimage and is not an indication that sex is wrong or bad. It is believed that by abstaining from sexual behavior, the person can focus all of their attention on the essence of the pilgrimage and not be distracted by other needs, wants, and desires. All of their emphasis and devotion is placed on the spiritual aspect of their lives for that specific allotment of time.

What could be helpful for many therapists to know is that following sexual intercourse, both men and women must perform full **ablution** before they may pray or touch or read the Qur'an. (Cohn-Sherbok et al., 2013, 44). An *ablution* is a religious ritual of washing. Once again, there are some similarities here to Judaism and ritual baths known as the *mikveh*. Within Islam, **ghusl** is also a ritual bath that involves washing the entire body (Fasasi, 2013), which is often performed whilst in the shower and is a relatively quick process. This is distinct from **wudū'**, which is a minor ablution for prayer (Salahi, 2020, 24).

Muslim Views on Sex Before Marriage

Cohen-Sherbok et al. (2013, 36) describe the topic of sexual morality within *shari'a* as untouchable. The majority of commentators agree that sex outside of marriage is completely forbidden. The term *zina*, refers to all sexual intercourse outside of the union between husband and wife and is similar to the English term "fornication." One common *āyah*, or verse, used to support this belief is 17:32, which states, "And come not near unto fornication. Lo! it is an abomination and an evil way."

Islamic law differs on what should happen to someone who commits fornication. It is written that, "the woman or man found guilty of adultery or fornication – lash each one of them with a hundred lashes, and do not be taken by pity for them in the religion of Allah, if you should believe in Allah and the Last Day. And let a group of the believers witness their punishment" (Quran 24:2). While this Quranic text mentions flogging as a punishment, there are several *hadiths* that mention stoning, including the *hadith* Sahih Bukhari – perhaps the most famous text outside of the Quran (Semerdjian, 2008, 8–14).

It is my opinion that the media often focuses on the most extreme cases in order to sensationalize stories and draw ratings. This is most definitely the case when dealing with topics related to religion or religious extremism. While it is true that there are cases in certain Middle Eastern countries where individuals have been stoned for their sexual behavior, one should not assume that this is the normal perspective of Islamic teaching. There are often differences in the *madhabs* that certain Islamic countries – such as Saudi Arabia – follow the more puritanical schools of thought, such as *wahhabism*. This is a good example of what was discussed in chapter one concerning the distinction between what a religious community (or, in this case, government) does and what the religious texts actually teach. In fact, for any disciplinary action to take place, it must be proved that fornication has transpired. Outside of a person confessing, it is rather difficult to establish such facts. *Shari'a* states that such an act must be exactly witnessed in the same way by four competent adult males or three men and two women – hearsay is not adequate and is discarded (Cohn-Sherbok et al., 2013, 37–38).

It can be easily reasoned that finding the appropriate witnesses to testify to the offense would be exceptionally difficult, if not impossible. While the position against premarital sex is strong, the position against false accusations of premarital sex is even stronger. The Quran states, "And those who accuse chaste women and then do not produce four witnesses – lash them with eighty lashes and do not accept from them testimony ever after. And those are the defiantly disobedient" (Quran 24:4). Therefore, the likelihood of such punishments being implemented is highly unlikely. The use of such language is done, as I explained in the chapter on Judaism, to emphasize the impact the person's behavior has on their spiritual well-being.

Muslim Views on Sex within Marriage

Marriage within Islam is of great importance. It is believed to be the foundation of society and the God-ordained institution for the formation of the family, as well as the environment best suited for the development of children (Cohn-Sherbok et al., 2013, 43). Interestingly, the Arabic word used for marriage, *nikah*, is also often translated as "sex." This should not be surprising considering the importance and value that Islam places on sexual interaction between husband and wife. Therefore, within the marital relationship, most sexual interactions are permissible and encouraged. For example, there are abundant Islamic texts on foreplay as being a necessary and crucial part of sexual intimacy, and that a husband should not leave his wife "hanging," so to speak, and to place her pleasure and fulfillment first (Al-Kawthari, 2015). Furthermore, the Quran states:

 Your wives are a tilth for you, so come to your place of cultivation however you wish and put forth [righteousness] for yourselves.

Quran 2:223

While the Quran does give permission to do "however you wish" between husband and wife, there are some prohibitions, even within marriage. For example, there should be no penetrating of the anus, no sex during menstruation, nor when it is harmful to the woman or if there is a valid reason from either spouse (Rassool & Khan, 2020, 106). Additionally, intercourse is not permitted during the 40 days following childbirth (Cohn-Sherbok et al., 2013, 44). Once again, these boundaries around sex should not be viewed as sex negative, but instead as a time for the female partner to focus on her well-being as well as the couple adjusting to the new addition to their family. Given that sex within marriage is a form of spiritual worship, and sexual pleasure a reflection of the afterlife, coercion or manipulation by either spouse is seen as counteracting the compassionate nature of marriage and going against one of the aims of the *shariah*, which is the sanctity and preservation of human life.

Muslim Views on Sex Outside of Marriage

Simply stated, Islam discourages sex outside of the marital relationship. This is true for both fornication and adultery. Fornication is thought of as sex between two people who are not married. Whereas adultery is also sex between two people who are not married to each other, however, one or both of the participants are married to someone else. Such behaviors are taken seriously.

Within Islamic law, there are mandatory punishments, known as *hudud*, for certain offenses. Included in those for capital punishment are illicit sex between married people and illicit sex between unmarried people or legal minors (Sonn, 2011, 53–54). However, as previously discussed, according to the Quran, in order for such penalties to be implemented, witnesses are required. Thus, the likelihood of severe punishment is minimal despite the harsh words recorded in the sacred text. Additionally, it should be noted that in these instances, the married person receives the maximum penalty, whereas the unmarried person receives the minimal penalty (Bouhdiba, 2012, 12). This places the greatest weight of the offense on the married party since their actions also affect their partner and family.

Muslim Views of Other Sexual Behaviors

As has been explored in the previous two chapters, there are other sexual behaviors besides penis and vaginal penetration that must be explored. Therefore, it is helpful to explore other sexual behaviors and the way that they are viewed within Islam. Once again, the topics of masturbation, homosexuality, and gender identity will be examined.

Masturbation

The topic of masturbation within Islamic teachings is one that elicits varying opinions among scholars and within Muslim communities. While there is no explicit mention of masturbation in the Quran, interpretations of hadith literature and Islamic jurisprudence offer guidance on the matter. The majority of Islamic scholars consider masturbation to be haram, meaning it is religiously forbidden. They base this perspective on the principle of preserving one's chastity and controlling one's desires in a manner consistent with Islamic teachings. They argue that sexual gratification should be sought within the bounds of a lawful marital relationship, and any form of sexual activity outside of that context is deemed sinful.

Some scholars, however, acknowledge certain exceptional circumstances where masturbation may be allowed or viewed as the lesser of two evils. For instance, if an individual is struggling with intense sexual urges and fears committing a more grievous offense, such as fornication or adultery, they may permit masturbation as a means of harm reduction. In such cases, it is seen as a pragmatic approach to prevent greater transgressions.

Nevertheless, it is important to note that the permissibility of masturbation in such exceptional circumstances remains a matter of debate among scholars, and opinions may vary. The consensus among the majority of scholars is that masturbation is discouraged or considered impermissible due to its potential negative consequences on one's spiritual and mental well-being.

Hadith literature, which consists of the sayings and actions of the prophet Muhammad, provides some guidance regarding the avoidance of masturbation. Certain hadiths highlight the importance of self-restraint, purity, and control over one's desires as fundamental aspects of leading a pious and disciplined life. These teachings emphasize the need to protect one's chastity and avoid actions that may lead to the indulgence of sexual desires outside of a lawful marital relationship.

It is worth noting that the issue of masturbation, like many other topics within Islamic teachings, is approached differently by different scholars and communities. Some may take a more lenient stance, considering it as a permissible act under certain circumstances, while others may adhere to a stricter interpretation and deem it entirely forbidden. Furthermore, it is important to address the practical aspect of masturbation within Islamic teachings. If an individual engages in masturbation, Islamic law requires them to perform ghusl, a ritual bath of purification. This is seen as a means to spiritually cleanse oneself after engaging in an act that is considered impure or sinful.

Overall, the topic of masturbation in Islam remains a complex and debated subject. While the majority of scholars consider it forbidden or strongly discouraged, there are differing opinions on its permissibility under exceptional circumstances. It is important for individuals seeking guidance on this matter to consult knowledgeable scholars, seek spiritual advice, and engage in self-reflection to navigate their personal beliefs and practices in accordance with their understanding of Islamic teachings.

There is a difference of opinion on the topic of masturbation – yet the most common conclusions often reached is that masturbation is *haraam*, or religiously impermissible, or that it is strongly discouraged, In fact, in some instances, masturbation is allowed as if it can stop the individual from committing a more grievous offense, like fornication or adultery. In such cases, masturbation can be considered the "lesser of two evils" and be allowed. Nevertheless, *hadith* literature gives detailed instructions on how avoiding masturbation is essential for living a pious life and it is considered **haram**, or forbidden, by the majority of scholars (Rassool & Khan, 2020, 161). Furthermore, an individual who masturbates must perform *ghusl*.

Oral Sex

The topic of oral sex within Islamic teachings is one that has generated differing opinions among scholars and within Muslim communities. While neither the Quran nor the hadith explicitly addresses the subject, scholars have offered varying interpretations regarding its permissibility within the context of the marital relationship. Scholars who argue for the permissibility of oral sex within marriage rely on certain legal principles and scholarly reasoning. They argue that as long as oral sex does not lead to the release of semen, it can be considered permissible. Some jurists, such as Al-Qaradawi, assert that both cunnilingus (oral stimulation of the female genitalia) and fellatio (oral stimulation of the male genitalia) are permissible within the bounds of marriage.

Neither the Quran nor the *hadith* specifically prohibit oral sex. Still, scholars are divided on whether or not oral sex is allowed within the marital relationship. According to Al-Qaradawi et al. (1980), Muslim jurists believe that it is lawful for both cunnilingus and fellatio to be performed as long as fellatio does not lead to the releasing of semen. In other words, the issue seems not to be the pleasure gained from kissing and licking the genitals but the possible ingestion of bodily fluids during fellatio, which Al-Nawawi (2016) describes as "disgusting (*mustakhbath*)."

Homosexuality

Within Islam, homosexuality is strictly forbidden. Cohn-Sherbok et al. (2013, 44) state that, "This is an absolute and there is no room for any argument for it to be permitted." Ramadan (2017, 185) concurs, pointing out, "The consensus of religious scholars, Sunni as well as Shi'a, is near unanimous. A number of questions have nonetheless been raised, dealing with differentiating between homosexual persons and homosexual acts, passive and active homosexuality (the latter being forbidden), female homosexuality (which is less frequently encountered but also forbidden in the literature), or the individual's right to a private life away from public view."

One of the primary texts found in the Quran that condemns male-on-male sexual activity states:

 And [We had sent] Lot when he said to his people, "Do you commit such immorality as no one has preceded you with from among the worlds? Indeed, you approach men with desire instead of women. Rather, you are a transgressing people." But the answer of his people was only that they said, "Evict them from your city! Indeed, they are men who keep themselves pure." So We saved him and his family, except for his wife; she was of those who remained [with the evildoers]. And We rained upon them a rain [of stones]. Then see how was the end of the criminals.

Quran 7:80–84

Similar to Judaism, the topic of lesbianism is viewed a bit differently than male-on-male sexual interactions. According to Myrne (2020, 147), "Sexual acts between two women are typically ruled on leniently, if mentioned at all. Some scholars believe this is due to the fact that it does not involve "penetration." Still, such behavior is considered a *haram* and there are scholars who do regard such behavior as a major sin though there is no *hadd* punishment. Therefore, it is not uncommon to see individuals of either gender who have same-sex attraction confused and unsure how to navigate their attraction with their religious beliefs.

Gender Identity

When it comes to the topic of gender identity, there is nothing specifically mentioned in the Quran or the *hadiths* concerning such topics as transsexuality or transgenderism. Much of the conversation surrounding Islam and gender identity depends on the prevailing thoughts of individual Muslim nations. Attitudes about transgenderism differ between governments, once again demonstrating how various communities interpret and apply sacred texts in different ways. For example, while the Iranian government is intolerant of homosexuality, it is more tolerant of transgenderism and permits gender reassignment procedures, which include changing the legal status of the individual. In fact, the government goes so far as to contribute to the cost of such procedures. Interestingly, there are reports that families have pressured their children to obtain gender reassignment procedures in order to avoid being accused of homosexuality and thus facing such consequences (Cohn-Sherbok et al., 2013, 46).

Conclusion

Sex within Islam plays a very essential role in the marital relationship. It is seen as a form of spiritual worship and reflective of the pleasures of the Afterlife, as an important vehicle whereby couples are able to connect physically and emotionally, as well as expand their family. Within the confines of the husband-wife relationship, most sexual activities are permissible and even encouraged by Islamic texts, with detailed texts available. Nevertheless, there are some boundaries that are primarily in place to protect both partners' physical health and well-being.

Outside of the marital relationship, Islam has many more boundaries concerning sexual relations. These areas include sex with oneself, sex with those of the same biological sex, and sex with those of the opposite biological gender. While these prohibitions may seem extreme to some, it is important to recognize the cultural and historical context in which these prohibitions are given and the spiritual wisdom behind such rulings. Additionally, it is important to recognize the additional stipulations given within the sacred texts concerning the application of punishment toward certain prohibited behaviors.

While it may be easy to focus on the boundaries that Islam places around certain sexual behaviors, it can be much more useful to focus on aspects that are helpful in the therapeutic setting, such as the often-overlooked texts which give protection to the female partner and focus on her well-being and the emphasis on familial relationships. Additionally, the view that the role of sex within the couples' relationship is connective, spiritual, sacred, special, and encouraged in Islam, is exceptionally beneficial when working through a number of sexual dysfunctions and difficulties that the couple may experience.

References

Al-Kawathari, M. I. A. (2015). *Islamic Guide to Sexual Relations*. Turath Publishing.

Al-Nawawi. (2016). *Kitab al-Majmu' Sharh al-Muhadhdhab*. DKI.

Al-Qaradawi, Y., El-Helbawy, K., & Qaraḍāwī, Y. (1980). *The Lawful and the Prohibited in Islam =: al-Halal wal-haram fīl Islam* (K. El-Helbawy & M. M. Siddiqui, Trans.). American Trust Publications.

Blair, S., & Bloom, J. (2002). *Islam: A Thousand Years of Faith and Power*. Yale University Press.

Bouhdiba, A. (2012). *Sexuality in Islam*. Saqi Books.

Cohn-Sherbok, D., Chryssides, G. D., & El Alami, D. S. (2013). *Love, Sex and Marriage: Insights from Judaism, Christianity and Islam*. SCM Press.

Fasasi, M. I. (2013). Ritual Bath in islam (Ghusl Janabat). *Ife Psychologia*, *21*(3), 72–74.

Haleem, M. A. S. A. (Trans.). (2008). *The Qur'an*. Oxford University Press.

Ibrahim, C. (2022). *Islam and Monotheism*. Cambridge University Press.

Kaltner, J. (2016). *Islam: What Non-Muslims Should Know* (J. Kaltner, Trans.). Fortress Press.

Mazokopakis, E. E. (2020). Sexual activity during menstruation in the Holy Bible and Quran. *International Journal of Fertility & Sterility*, *14*(1), 78. DOI: 10.22074/ijfs.2020.6060

Muhammad, G. B. (2017). *A thinking Persons Guide to Islam: The Essence of Islam in Twelve Verses from the Quran*. White Thread Press.

Myrne, P. (2020). *Female Sexuality in the Early Medieval Islamic World: Gender and Sex in Arabic Literature* (R. Mottahedeh, Ed.). Bloomsbury Academic.

Peters, F. E. (2018). *The Children of Abraham: Judaism, Christianity, Islam*. Princeton University Press.

Ramadan, T. (2017). *Introduction to Islam*. Oxford University Press.

Rassool, G. H., & Khan, M. A. (2020). *Sexuality Education from an Islamic Perspective*. Cambridge Scholars Publishing.

Salahi, A. (Ed.). (2020). *Sahih Muslim (Volume 3): With the Full Commentary by Imam Nawawi* (A. Salahi, Trans.). Islamic Foundation.

Semerdjian, E. (2008). *"Off the Straight Path": Illicit Sex, Law, and Community in Ottoman Aleppo*. Syracuse University Press.

Sonn, T. (2011). *Islam: A Brief History*. Wiley.

PART III

Working with Religious Patients through Sexual Issues

Overview

Drawing upon the knowledge and skills introduced in the preceding sections, the forthcoming part of this text will center its attention on the practical implementation of these concepts in a clinical setting. Within each chapter, we will delve into the typical challenges faced by religious patients in the context of psychosexual therapy, elucidating effective approaches that honor and align with their religious beliefs and perspectives.

Learning Objectives

- ♦ Identify differences in approach when working with Jewish, Christian, and Muslim patients presenting with the same issue.
- ♦ Recognize areas of bias when working with religious patients on specific psychosexual issues.
- ♦ Apply the steps in the Jacobson model to use when working with religious patients.
- ♦ Recall important religious principles that can impact the therapeutic alliance.

DOI: 10.4324/9781003242017-10

7

Masturbation and Porn

Introduction

While specific attitudes regarding masturbation vary depending on the person's religious background, in general, masturbation is typically not encouraged,[1] and in most cases it is blatantly discouraged. This does not mean that religious individuals do not masturbate, similar to the general population, it is not uncommon to find that many do. While some religious individuals have found congruence between their decision to masturbate and the teachings of their faith tradition, many religious patients do struggle with anxiety, guilt, and shame associated with masturbation. These feelings become even greater when pornography is used in conjunction with masturbation.

All three Abrahamic faiths condemn the use of pornographic material, and many religious individuals who view pornography state it troubles their conscience as it violates their religious beliefs (Hoagland et al., 2023). It is not surprising, then, that it is through the lens of religion that the term addiction has been inappropriately applied to problematic uses of pornography[2] (Neves, 2021). Incidentally, research has long indicated that pornography has the greatest negative impact on religious individuals (Patterson & Price, 2012; Perry & Whitehead, 2019). Therefore, a religious person self-describing addiction to porn and masturbation addiction is not uncommon. In the following case studies, we

DOI: 10.4324/9781003242017-11

will view instances where porn and masturbation have impacted religiously observant individuals and couples.

Therapist Bias Check

1. In your opinion, how important is the role of masturbation to a person's sexual health?
2. How comfortable are you being challenged about your beliefs concerning the morality of porn?

Case Study 1 – Nathan

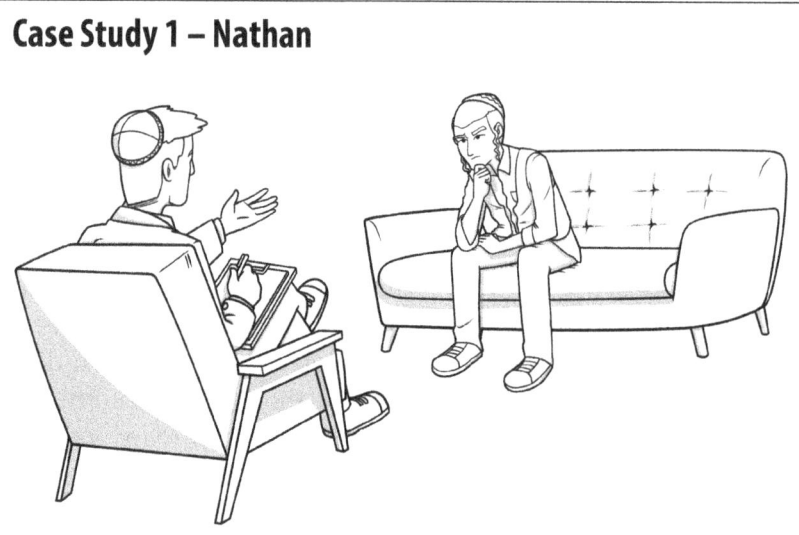

Uri is a 20-year-old Yeshivah student who is struggling with what he believes is an addiction to masturbation. Although he knows that it is considered wrong in his community, he finds himself masturbating two or three times a week. He worries that this behavior will prevent him from getting married and affect his sexual relationship with his future spouse. Uri also fears that others will find out about his addiction and that it will prevent him from receiving *smicha*, or rabbinical ordination. Despite trying to stop on his own, Uri has been unsuccessful and now feels overwhelmed by guilt, shame, and a sense of failure. He has come to therapy seeking help to stop masturbating and to alleviate his negative emotions.

Initial Interaction

During the first interactions with Nathan, it was apparent he was nervous. He was a bit fidgety and seemed uncomfortable, even with initial introductions and small talk. With most religious patients, I introduce myself and mention my qualifications in both psychology and biblical studies, often adding a statement like, "so I'm looking forward to working with you as I feel that we will both come from a place of similar understanding." From there, the Permission element of the PLISSIT model is introduced. I stated to Nathan, "I always like to begin my sessions by asking for permission to discuss really personal sexual topics, will that be alright with you?" To which he responded, "yes." I continued by saying, "I also want to use this time for you to give yourself permission to discuss sexual topics as well. I know that sometimes it's awkward or uncomfortable, but I want you to feel safe and liberated in this space to do so, okay?" To which he nodded and replied, "Thank you."

Step 1 – Identify

Following the initial introduction, the foundational step in the therapeutic process invariably entails the precise identification of the presenting issue. In Nathan's case, this crucial aspect became unequivocally evident during the initial assessment phase. His primary motivation for seeking therapy was explicitly linked to the need to gain mastery over his masturbatory habits. Nathan held an unwavering conviction that his life was being grievously compromised by his engagement in masturbation, laboring under the misguided belief that by exerting control over this impulse and refraining from it, his life would undergo a transformative improvement.

Step 2 – Uncover

Subsequently, a paramount consideration lay in the meticulous examination of the underlying reasons for the profound challenge posed by masturbation in Nathan's case. Distinct from non-religious patients, whose struggles with masturbation might stem from influences such as family upbringing, media exposure, or peer pressure, Nathan's predicament was intrinsically intertwined with the ideological messaging propagated by his faith community. In Nathan's worldview, the imperative to cease masturbation stemmed directly from the deeply ingrained religious doctrines that framed his beliefs about this practice. Within the tenets of Orthodox Judaism, any sexual act culminating in ejaculation outside the vaginal context is deemed to be in contravention of religious teachings, thereby necessitating avoidance.

Step 3 – Recognize

The traditional teaching of Orthodox Judaism pertaining to masturbation appears to stand in stark contrast to the tenets typically promoted within the realm of sexual health, thereby presenting a potential source of bias for the practitioner. It becomes imperative for the clinician to conscientiously reflect upon the ways in which the patient's perspectives on masturbation and pornography may directly challenge their own established beliefs and, in turn, engender a fundamental discordance within the therapeutic alliance. This consideration underscores the crucial importance of self-awareness and the proactive management of potential biases in the therapeutic process.

Step 4 – Develop

After identifying both the presenting problem and the underlying religious factors contributing to it, the determination of the most appropriate course of action to help Nathan reconcile his religious beliefs with his sexual behavior was attainable. As a clinician committed to the principle of not imposing personal beliefs on those I work with, my role is to challenge the thoughts and behaviors of my patients while refraining from influencing their choices based on my own moral compass. In Nathan's case, he confronted three distinct options: (1) maintaining abstinence from masturbation in alignment with his religious convictions, (2) abandoning his religious values in favor of unrestricted masturbation, or (3) embarking on a journey to deepen his comprehension of both his religious and sexual values, thus prompting a reevaluation of his perspective on masturbation.

The first option posed inherent challenges, as Nathan's previous attempts in this direction had culminated in distress, anxiety, guilt, and shame, ultimately leading him to therapy. The second option also proved problematic, as forsaking his deeply held religious beliefs would be incongruent with his authentic self and likely lead to future regrets. Conversely, by undertaking the endeavor of enhancing his understanding of the interplay between his religious and sexual values, Nathan could make well-informed decisions grounded in empirical insights, fostering spiritual and personal growth in the process.

The path to congruency always begins with **psychosexual education**. I asked Nathan what he thought and knew about masturbation. His knowledge of the topic of masturbation was dismal. He knew the basic technique of masturbation and knew that his religious tradition discouraged the practice. I began by showing him a diagram of the male anatomy, explaining that it was important for him to understand his own body and that this knowledge would also be beneficial in the future when he had a sexual partner. I then asked him if he understood how sex works; meaning penis to vagina intercourse. To which he replied he had some idea. Therefore, I was able to present him with some basic education on conjugal relations. This opened up the door for me to discuss the emotional, psychological, and physical benefits of sex.

After discussing the benefits of sex, I began to explain how many of the same benefits are achieved through masturbation. I even incorporated some empirical evidence to support a reduction in stress levels, improved sleep, and the less likelihood of developing prostate cancer. This information was very compelling for him as he began to understand the health benefits associated with sexual functioning, as well as understanding that masturbation has positive components. This challenges his belief that masturbation is inherently bad and detrimental to a person's overall well-being while helping him to establish his own sexual values.

Next, it was time to **incorporate some of his faith tradition** into the therapeutic process. This begins by simply asking Nathan, "How does your religious beliefs inform the way that you think about masturbation?" This is the time for me to challenge Nathan on what his religion teaches about masturbation. The goal is not to have him abandon what his religion teaches about masturbation but to have him actually consider if he accepts those teachings himself or if he simply does it because he feels he must.

Nathan stated that he knew masturbation was wrong because of the story of Onan found in Genesis 38:8–10. I didn't begin to question him as to his understanding of the biblical text. It was very clear to me that his interpretation was void of many cultural variables presented in the text and references in other biblical passages. So I gave Nathan homework. His homework assignment was to examine the Onan narrative and discover what other commentators, scholars, and rabbis have thought and written about the text. The goal was not to change his religious conviction; instead, it was to allow him to begin to think more critically about the text.

After spending time studying the text, Nathan noticed that the issue within the biblical narrative had nothing to do with masturbation. While this was a major progression in the therapeutic process, it didn't mean that he automatically was fine with masturbating. He still faced hurdles surrounding Jewish law and his communities' traditions. Additionally, I still had concerns over his relationship with masturbation and wanted Nathan to begin to explore the way he felt about his sexual behavior with himself. This led to the third step of **finding creative solutions**.

It was necessary to help Nathan establish a sense of self-identity and to have some autonomy over his sexuality. This does not mean that he has to abandon his community's boundaries, but it does mean that he needs to make a conscious and empowering decision. This way, regardless of what he chooses, he will be empowered by his decision. I started by asking two questions:

- *Are you comfortable having different opinions than that of your religious community?*
- *What do you personally think about masturbation?*

In analyzing the first question, it was clear that the patient needed to develop a more confident sense of self. The entirety of his identity was enveloped in his community. While I advocate for strong communal ties, I also recognize that it is important for a person to have individualism. It is within the friction of collectivism and individualism that people are able to grow, develop, and flourish as they find fulfillment in all areas of their personhood. This led to a series of sessions simply discussing Nathan's likes, dislikes, interests, and thoughts. It was equally as important to understand how he felt about certain things in his life. This provided him an opportunity to critically contemplate areas of his life that he never considered before and gave him permission to explore the intersection of his thoughts and feelings.

After a few sessions focused on helping Nathan develop a sense of self-identity, I then raised the question of masturbation. In reflection of the early psychosexual education session and his study of the biblical texts, Nathan asserted his belief that masturbation was not forbidden in the biblical text and acknowledged that masturbation did have some physical and psychological benefits if done in moderation. He did state that despite these feelings, he wanted to live within the boundaries that his religious community placed on masturbation. To him, it was important to observe and live within that tradition.

Focus in therapy then began to focus on his personal masturbation habits. It was important for me that Nathan began to think about his own acts and discover how he felt about them after his cognitive shift. Questions were raised, such as: "How will you reconcile self-pleasure from time to time with your choice to observe your faith traditions abstinence from masturbation?" To this question, he responded that his choice not to masturbate was his own. He stated that he was keeping that boundary because he wanted to, not because he was told to. His answers demonstrated that he was taking autonomy over his sexual behavior.

Final sessions with Nathan focused on his fear of people knowing he masturbated. In this session, he appeared to be far more relaxed than in earlier sessions. I asked, "So what would you do now if someone did catch you masturbating?" Nathan laughed for a minute and then responded, "I guess I would ask them what are they doing watching me?" It appeared that the previous fear had lost intensity but further inquiry was made to ensure the patient fully contemplated the situation. The question was posed, "How would you respond then if people found out that you masturbated?" He replied, "I would tell them I don't feel that law is based in the Torah, and while I choose to uphold it most of the time, sometimes I don't and I'm okay with that." He then added, "And it's really none of their business."

Ultimately, Nathan decided that his convictions about masturbation were not as strong as he originally thought. He decided that he personally did not think masturbation was problematic but wanted to try and honor his faith tradition by adhering to its teachings on masturbation to the best of his ability. He reported that he still masturbated on occasion but no longer felt anxiety about his decision to do so.

Case Study 2 – Allison

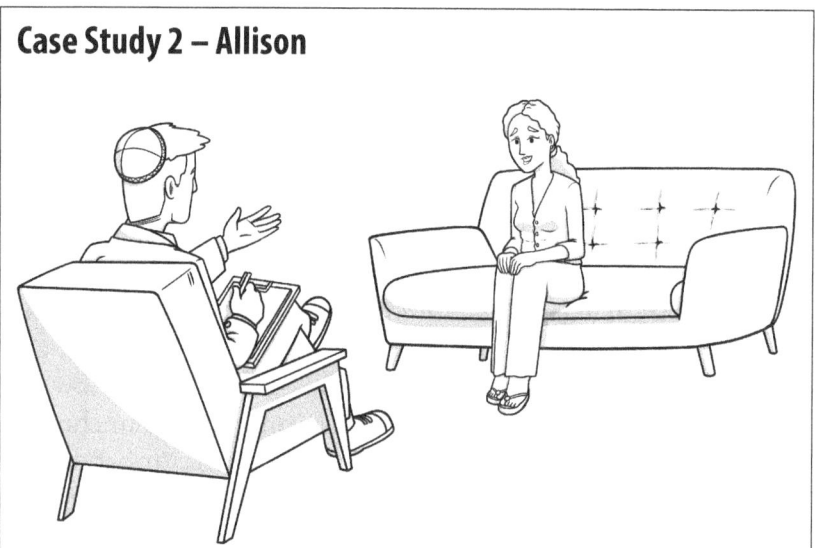

Allison is a 19-year-old Christian who belongs to a charismatic church. She came to therapy due to attempted suicide. She is severely depressed because she is unable to control her desire to masturbate. She states that her addiction to masturbation is so bad that she must first masturbate before she is able to go to sleep at night. She has tried numerous methods to stop masturbating but to no avail. During a recent revival service, Allison went to the front of her church to repent of her "lustful thoughts and perverse actions." She later confessed to her youth pastor that she has a problem with masturbation and has been unable to stop, no matter how hard she tries. Allison's youth pastor told her that she must be struggling with a demon. That evening they asked her to come to the front of the church to have the demon "cast out" of her. She described the experience as being very intense. She says after members of the church "laid hands" on her and prayed to cast out the demon, she felt free and liberated from the desire to pleasure herself. However, the desire to masturbate returned a few weeks later. Feeling defeated and overwhelmed, Allison felt the only way to overcome these feelings was to try and end her own life.

Initial Interaction

When Allison presented for the first time, she seemed almost lifeless. She was experiencing extreme hopelessness and felt that therapy was just a waste of time. She described that she had completely given up on life and saw no reason to continue living. As she continuously avoided direct conversation and discussion concerning masturbation, it was obvious that she was avoidant of using the term and felt that such discussions would even be considered evil and wrong. Due to this mental framework, it was important to reiterate and re-emphasize the permission aspect of the PLISSIT model. Simply asking Allison to give herself permission to discuss sexual things one time would not have been enough to solidify in her subconscious that such discussions were allowed, much less useful to her situation.

Step 1 – Identify

Allison's initial clinical presentation was unequivocal in its gravity. She grappled with a profound and debilitating depression, compounded by recurring suicidal ideation. Her pervasive sense of hopelessness had led her to abandon any semblance of purpose in life.

Step 2 – Uncover

There were two areas in which Allison's religious beliefs impacted her condition. While the views on masturbation within the evangelical movement may be ambiguous, depending on the denomination, the position the movement has taken on pornography is not. Allison did not describe it as her primary issue. When I asked her during the assessment if she used pornography, she admitted that she did, although she stated she only used it 30% of the time. In her mind, she was not masturbating because she was watching porn. She was watching porn because she was masturbating. Therefore she believed that if she could control her masturbation, then she would not need to think about porn consumption any longer. Nevertheless, she had great guilt and shame over her masturbatory behavior and the use of pornography.

As she was unable to control either of these, she began having severe internal conflicts, which caused depression. It is very common within evangelical Christian groups to confuse mental illness with demonic activity or sin (Lloyd, 2021). In this case, her church declared she was demonically possessed. However, when prayer and the casting out of demonic spirits did not work, Allison's self-worth and self-esteem were greatly diminished since the lack of "deliverance" from demonic activity and sin could only mean that God did not care about her. This is in line with recent research showing the negative impact that belief in demons has on a person's mental health (Nie & Olson, 2016).

Step 3 – Recognize

When Allison first disclosed her story, I was troubled by the treatment she had received from her church. I strongly felt that the behavior was abusive and the cause for a large percentage of the distress that she was trying to cope with. However, since faith was such a big part of Allison's life, I needed to ensure that my bias did not interfere with the therapeutic alliance. In order to do that, I mainly focused our discussions around the texts that she held sacred and not the actions or beliefs of her particular community.

Step 4 – Develop

When asked about her suicide attempt, Allison stated that she was going to go to hell for masturbating, and then, while she cannot control the length of eternity, she can control the length of time that she was in hell on earth. It was clear from that statement that she was going through severe mental anguish. She frequently mentioned that she would never be free from her "addiction" to masturbation. This provided a wonderful opportunity to begin with **psychosexual education.**

Allison had gone to a Christian high school where she never received any sex education. All of the information she learned about sex came from the internet and from absence-based messages she heard in church. One particular event she recalls is a three-day youth and family retreat that her church held where they brought in speakers, including teenage and early college-aged, to discuss abstinence. She recognized this event as being extremely impactful to her spiritually and in the formation of her thoughts and values around sex.

As we began education around sex, I covered common themes about anatomy, sexual functioning, and the role of sex as being both for procreation and for pleasure. Due to her religious background, it was important for me to frame the discussion about pleasure within the context of the marital relationship. This allowed her to accept the information without feeling offended or that she needed to offer an apologetic to what I was sharing. It also allowed me to pose the following question: Why do you think God made a connection between sex and pleasure?

This question led us to the second step of **incorporating the faith tradition** into the therapeutic process. Allison shared that she believed God connected pleasure and sex so that couples would have more intimate times together since it feels so good. This reflection was important as it started building a connection between sex and pleasure in Allison's mind. After her response, I asked, "So God made our bodies to feel pleasure?" She nodded in agreement. "Would you say it's a good thing that our bodies can feel pleasure?" She once again indicated that she thought it was good. I did not antagonize the patient by asking a question such as, "Then why does God not want you to feel pleasure on your own?" This would have been problematic, causing the patient to close down and become defensive. Instead, I switched to the topic of emotional pain by asking, "Do you believe God wants you to be happy?" Once again, Allison said, "yes."

The patient's responses demonstrated an inconsistency. On one hand, she states that she feels God has abandoned her, on the other, she states that she believes God wants her to be happy. Here is where it is possible to use the benefits of religion, primarily as it relates to optimism and purpose, to help overcome Allison's cognitive dissonance. This is where we began to find **creative solutions** to find congruence in two areas:

1. Perceptions of what God thinks about her.
2. Perceptions of what God thinks about pleasure.

Regarding the first point, it was suspected that a source of Allison's depression was her perception that God did not care about her. This was something that affected her greatly, given that her Charismatic background emphasized a strong personal relationship with God. However, due to the lack of "deliverance" that she experienced during the exorcism, Allison felt that she had been abandoned by God and that he had turned his back on her.

The plan was to help Allison rethink her relationship with God and avoid the faulty cognitions that she possessed concerning that relationship. It was believed that by doing so, it would help to reduce her distress, improve her mood, and give her the motivation needed to find congruency concerning her sexual behavior. This plan allowed for further incorporation of Allison's faith tradition in the therapeutic process. Over the course of four weeks, Allison was told to meditate on certain Bible verses as her homework. During the following session, questions surrounding the verses were raised in order to help facilitate further thought and overcome her fear of abandonment.

Week One

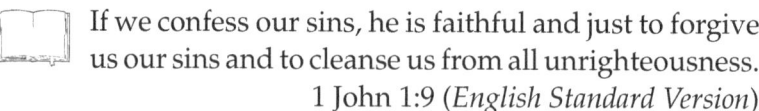

If we confess our sins, he is faithful and just to forgive us our sins and to cleanse us from all unrighteousness.

1 John 1:9 (*English Standard Version*)

◆ *What does this verse mean?*

"This verse means that God will always forgive us, no matter what we do, if we confess our sins to him because Jesus gave his life on the cross for us."

- ♦ *According to this verse, if you confess your sins to God, will he forgive you?*

"Yes."

- ♦ *Do you normally confess your sins when you feel you have done something sinful?*

"Yes, I even asked God to forgive me of sins that I didn't know I committed as well."

- ♦ *Then God has forgiven you?*

"Yes, God forgives everyone who asks him."

- ♦ *But each time you confess your sins?*

"Yeah."

- ♦ *Is there a limit on God's grace and mercy?*

"No, I don't believe so."

- ♦ *So would it be safe to assume you haven't reached that limit then, since there isn't one?*

"Yeah, that's true."

- ♦ *So who has given up? Has God given up on you or have you given up on God?*

"I don't know. But I guess, it seems to be me because I know that the Bible says God will never give up on me and he'll always forgive me."

Week Two

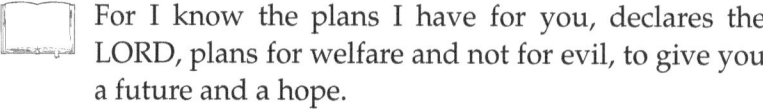 For I know the plans I have for you, declares the LORD, plans for welfare and not for evil, to give you a future and a hope.

Jeremiah 29:11 (*English Standard Version*)

◆ *What does this verse mean?*

"This verse means that God has a purpose for all of our lives, and that his plans are for our good, not for our bad."

◆ *Do you believe God has plans for your life?*

"Well, I used to always think so."

◆ *Do those plans include doing something evil to you?*

"No, of course not."

◆ *How do you know?*

"Because the verse says that his plans aren't for evil, but that he wants to give us a future and a hope."

◆ *But you said that God has abandoned you, or am I not understanding correctly?*

"No, I know I said that but I just felt really alone, although I know God wants good things for me and has a purpose for my life."

◆ *Can you think of any examples in the Bible where people felt that God abandoned them, but in actuality, he hadn't?*

"Yeah, I can think of a few. Elijah, in the Old Testament, was depressed because he felt God had abandoned him. And then Jesus on the cross asked God why he had forsaken him. And I would guess Paul felt abandoned too when he was shipwrecked."

◆ *Why do you think God did that?*

"I think God was testing their faith."

♦ *So, in the future, could it be possible for you to discover that God hasn't abandoned you but this was all a lesson to help you grow in your faith?*

"It could be, but it just doesn't like that right now. Like it is all hopeless."

♦ *What does Jeremiah 29:11 say about that?*

"It says that God's plans are for my future and that there is hope."

Week Three

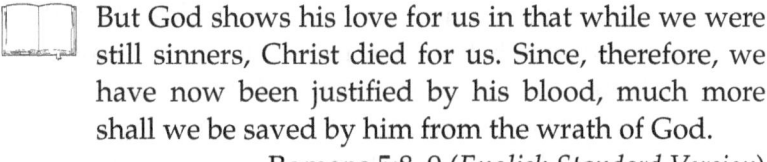 But God shows his love for us in that while we were still sinners, Christ died for us. Since, therefore, we have now been justified by his blood, much more shall we be saved by him from the wrath of God.

Romans 5:8–9 (*English Standard Version*)

♦ *What does this verse mean?*

"It means that Jesus died for our sins when we were sinners, and they will be saved."

♦ *The first part of the verse says God loved you while you were a sinner, or am I misinterpreting it?*

"No, that's correct."

♦ *Did God love you while you sinned before you were a Christian?*

"Yes."

♦ *So while you were a sinner and doing sinful things, God loved you?*

"Yes."

◆ *So why does God stop loving Christians if they sin? Wouldn't it be better to never be a Christian so that God will love you when you are sinning?*

"No, God does still love all of us even if we sin, and that's why we must confess our sins, so who continue to forgive us even after we become Christians."

◆ *Oh, then why don't you think God loves you?*

"He just feels like he doesn't sometimes because I feel like I keep messing up. But I know deep inside he really does love me."

Week Four

 Who shall separate us from the love of Christ? Shall tribulation, or distress, or persecution, or famine, or nakedness, or danger, or sword? As it is written, "For your sake we are being killed all the day long; we are regarded as sheep to be slaughtered." No, in all these things we are more than conquerors through him who loved us. For I am sure that neither death nor life, nor angels nor rulers, nor things present nor things to come, nor powers, nor height nor depth, nor anything else in all creation, will be able to separate us from the love of God in Christ Jesus our Lord.

Romans 8:35–38 (*English Standard Version*)

◆ *What does this verse mean?*

"It means that Jesus is always gonna love us, no matter what we do, and that nothing can come between us and the love of God."

◆ *So according to what you're telling me God will always love you no matter what?*

"Yes, it even mentions a bunch of things like tribulation, Life, and death."

◆ *And nothing that could ever happen, or nothing that you could ever do could separate you from that?*

"Right."

◆ *What if you lie? Would God still love you?*

"Yes, God still loves me."

◆ *And if you, move to some God-forsaken place like Arkansas, would God still love you?*

"Well I wouldn't move there but yes, God would still love me if I did."

◆ *What if you masturbate this afternoon, would God still love you?*

"Yeah, I guess so."

◆ *So you recognize that God will still love you, but earlier, you said you felt that he had abandoned you. It seems like the real issue is there is a disconnect between your thoughts and your actions, not so much if God actually loves you or not, would you agree?*

"Yeah, that's right."

As I worked through the scenarios with Allison, it became clear that she began to recognize that the issue was not that God had abandoned her, but that she had a disconnect between her desire, not to masturbate based upon her religious beliefs, and the fact that she had urges that she met through masturbation. At this point in the therapeutic process, Allison admitted that her mood had improved and that she had begun spending time praying and listening to religious music every day. She stated that she felt very good about these decisions and felt it was a move in the right direction. I inquired concerning her masturbation routine and discovered that she was still masturbating regularly. She mentioned that this most commonly happened at night as she was falling asleep.

The second perception where Allison had cognitive dissonance was concerning what God thinks about pleasure. This was the underlying issue in her disconnect between her thoughts about masturbation and her beliefs about masturbation. For this work, I intentionally digressed from dealing with the topic of pornography. If necessary, this would have been a factor that I could have come back to discuss with the patient if needed. However, what was imperative, was to apply some of the psychosexual education that was conducted around masturbation to help Allison understand that she was not the victim of demonic possession.

The psychosexual education that was conducted covered the benefits of masturbation, including the reduction of stress, the ability to help a person relax, and improved quality of sleep. From there, it was possible to draw a connection between her desire to masturbate as she was falling asleep, not to lustful thoughts, but to the self-care attributes of self-pleasure. Again, this is why I did not engage in discussion around pornography, as this was not the primary cause of the patient's distress, and their pornography use was infrequent.

After helping, Allison understand the connection between her masturbation and sleep, I didn't ask her what are some other ways that she could help to reduce some stress and relax before falling asleep. This is not because I want her to refrain from masturbation altogether, but I wanted to continue to reduce stress around the subject, in order to demonstrate that she had control over her sexual behavior. She listed a few alternatives, such as listening to music or sleep stories before bed. Therefore, we set up a regimented schedule around her sleep, where she would shower, brush her teeth, get in bed by 10:30 p.m., and would listen to either music or a sleep story. After trying this for a month, the patient reported that this was effective and that she was no longer masturbating before falling asleep.

Now that the patient felt that they had control over their masturbation habits, it was time to discuss Allison's values around sexual pleasure. This allowed me to revisit previous discussions that I had with Allison concerning the purposes of sex and if God intended for people to experience pleasure during sexual activity. No longer under the distress and faulty cognition concerning her masturbatory behavior, Allison was much more confident in stating that she believed that God intended sexual behavior to be pleasurable. I've been provided some additional psychosexual education concerning how arousal works, and the neurobiological processes that are connected with our sexual desire. While I allowed Allison, to ask questions concerning the information that I was sharing with her, I was ultimately able to ask her a very important question: "Why would God create our bodies to function a certain way, to feel good, and be programmed with certain desires if they were all bad?"

Allison stated that those feelings and desires were not bad or sinful if they are done within the right context. This led to the discussion around sexual boundaries where Allison was questioned about her sexual boundaries and values. She stated that she wasn't sure if masturbation was wrong or sinful, but it felt wrong because it felt so good. I then posed the question, "So it is wrong because it feels pleasurable, the way that God intended?" This question really made Allison stop and think.

The next week, Allison came to therapy stating that she had made some decisions. She stated that she didn't think that masturbation was wrong. However, she did want to avoid masturbating while looking at pornography, and she did not want to do it every night in order to fall asleep. It was then that I inquired about her sleep routine that we had begun three months ago. She informed me that she was still not masturbating to fall asleep but she did want alternatives to pornography.

It was important to understand exactly how Allison defined pornography. Within certain conservative groups, pornography is not just used to refer to photographs or videos containing nudity, but it could also refer to images of people and undergarments or books detailing sexually explicit encounters. For Allison, it was very simple: she defined pornography as sexually explicit imagery in both photos and videos. Therefore, I suggested that she begin to listen to audio erotica whenever she felt the urge to masturbate. I also inquired concerning her feelings about the use of a vibrator, to which she had some hesitation.

The idea behind the incorporation of the vibrator was that the patient would no longer use their hand to masturbate thus creating a distance between their physical touch and their experience of pleasure. For some religious patients whom I have worked with, this has reduced their anxiety around masturbation. However, in this case, when the patient was uncertain, I did not press the issue. Instead, I gave her a list of recommendations for audio erotica and suggested that she start with a free trial of multiple sources in order to find the one that she best connects with and feels the most comfortable with.

After seven months of working with Allison, she reported that she was no longer suicidal. While she still had some bad days, she felt very confident in her relationship with God, and cited it as one of the sources of her strength. She continued the practice of listening to music or sleep stories as she went to sleep each night. It was also clear that she had begun to develop a healthy relationship with her sexuality. She reported that she was masturbating 2 to 3 times a week on average, however, she did not feel bad or guilty. When masturbating, she stated that she would listen to audio erotica and commented that it opened the door to discovering what she likes sexually.

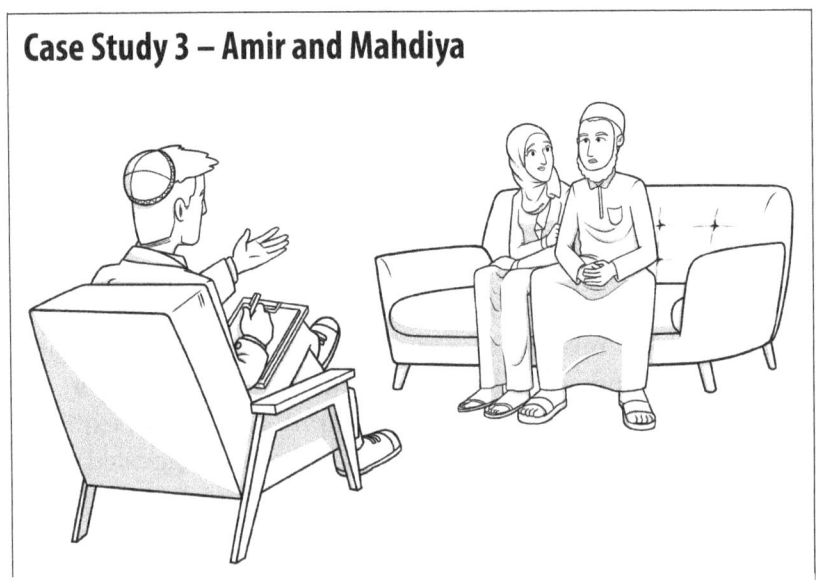

Case Study 3 – Amir and Mahdiya

Amir, a 30-year-old Muslim man, has been married to his wife, Mahdiya for 5 years. Recently, Mahdiya caught him watching porn and masturbating, which led to a heated discussion. She accused him of cheating on her and lying to her, which left Amir feeling ashamed and guilty. Amir admits to being addicted to porn and masturbation and acknowledges that it has impacted his relationship with Mahdiya. She is no longer interested in engaging in sexual activities with him until he addresses his issues. Amir is seeking help to overcome his porn usage and rebuild trust with his wife.

Initial Interaction

Upon first seeing the couple, it was apparent that communication had significantly deteriorated between them. Both seemed hurt and alone, lacking the skills to initiate a conversation with each other. During the initial intake, they were defensive and reactive, easily triggered by the other's comments. They both appeared conflicted Amir was completely confused. Even though he felt bad about masturbation because of his religious beliefs, he did not think he had an addiction, but his wife kept telling him that he did. Mahdiya was totally conflicted, on one hand, she felt totally betrayed by Amir and on the other, wanted to desperately help him as she truly believed he was dealing with an addiction that was beyond his control. The early sessions were tense, and any misstep could trigger an argument between the two. Yet, it was obvious that their religious faith was the primary reason that they both were willing to come to therapy.

The session began with the PLISSIT model, which involves asking for **P**ermission to discuss sexual topics and asking related questions. Both partners agreed to this. However, when they were both asked to give themselves permission to discuss sex as well, Mahdiya seemed hesitant. When probed further, she explained that she was worried about saying something that might make her husband look bad and that he was actually a good man. To address her concerns, I asked Amir if he would give Mahdiya permission to express herself freely in therapy, which he agreed to. This helped to alleviate some of her hesitation and made her more comfortable moving forward in the session.

Step 1 – Identify

Amir and Mahdiya are facing significant challenges in their relationship due to Amir's use of pornography. Mahdiya views this as an addiction and as a form of infidelity. As a result, she has refused to engage in any sexual interactions with her husband. This has created a sense of betrayal and mistrust between the couple, as Mahdiya feels that Amir has broken her trust and violated the boundaries of their marriage. There has been an extreme breakdown in communication. As such, the couple is experiencing a significant strain on their relationship, and they are seeking help to address these challenges. They are both committed to working through their problems and restoring their relationship, but they recognize that it will take time and effort to overcome the trust and intimacy issues.

Step 2 – Uncover

In Islam, both pornography usage and masturbation are considered to be undesirable behaviors. This helps to explain Amir's guilt and shame attached to his association with these areas. The use of pornography is seen as a violation of Islamic teachings on modesty and chastity (Alli, 2011, 24–25). It is viewed as a form of adultery, as it involves a person engaging in sexual thoughts and acts outside of marriage (Rassool & Khan, 2020). This explains why Mahdiya is convinced that Amir has cheated on her by viewing pornographic images. Additionally, Islamic scholars and leaders have spoken out against the use of pornography and masturbation, warning that they can lead to addiction, damage to relationships, and spiritual harm, informing her opinion that Amir has a pornography addiction.

Step 3 – Recognize

There were a number of possible ethical dilemmas that could arise when working with Amir and Mahdiya. First, due to their religious beliefs, it was necessary to avoid offering solutions that could violate the couple's convictions. In other words, I wouldn't recommend that they watch porn together. Second, since Mahdiya held to the notion of porn addiction, it was important for me to address my thoughts on the topic in an educational and informative way that was respectful of her position. I typically address the situation the following way:

> *I know you mentioned porn addiction. As we get started, I just want to be clear that I understand that there may be a problem with porn consumption, but as a clinician, I do not hold to the theory of porn addiction. This is primarily because I have found that an addiction model of treatment is not effective in treating these issues. This is in line with much of the current research and with the DSM-5, which is the diagnostic manual for the American Psychological Association.*

By explaining the situation to the patient in this way, it validates their feelings that there is an issue with porn consumption, but also moves the conversation away from discussions about addiction. By acknowledging their concern that there could be a problem, they are willing to listen to the professional recommendation and assessment from the provider. Additionally, as the provider it clarifies your professional stance to avoid any misunderstandings by allowing the patient to move forward under possible false pretenses.

Step 4 – Develop

Islam, similar to Judaism and Christianity, which has numerous limitations when it comes to sex education (Rassool & Khan, 2020, 179–180). This is why it is very important to begin the therapeutic alliance with **psychosexual education**. In this particular case, it was important for me to address the issue of addiction early on in the process. I explained to the couple that I did not follow an addiction model of treatment for porn usage, that pornography addiction is not included in the DSM-5, and that I did not find addiction treatment to be effective in such cases. Further, I explained that I was not saying there was an absence of problems related to porn consumption but that addiction was not the lens in which we would be addressing those issues.

The discussion surrounding addiction is of paramount significance for several compelling reasons. Firstly, it serves as a pivotal step towards dispelling any misconceptions the patients may hold regarding issues related to pornography consumption. To be candid, in a majority of my work with religious patients, the primary concern regarding their consumption of pornography lies in its contradiction with their religious convictions. However, there are instances where patients exhibit patterns of out-of-control sexual behavior or sexual compulsions, where pornography becomes a component of the issue.

Secondly, it's noteworthy that patients often respond with a heightened sense of optimism when the clinician elucidates their stance on pornography addiction. This effect is twofold: firstly, it conveys that the clinician has attentively acknowledged the patient's concerns and recognizes their significance; secondly, by articulating their expertise on the subject, the clinician instills a sense of confidence and reassurance in the religious patient. This, in turn, fosters a more relaxed and comfortable atmosphere within the therapeutic process.

Given that pornography was a primary area of concern, my initial objective was to gain a comprehensive understanding of both partners' perspectives on pornography. Mahdiya forthrightly expressed her belief that pornography was morally reprehensible, equating it to infidelity and feeling betrayed by Amir's consumption. She also contended that pornography was degrading to women. On the other hand, Amir acknowledged certain ethical concerns associated with pornography but did not view it as tantamount to infidelity. However, he did consider it morally wrong based on his religious beliefs.

Masturbation was also an area where I felt it was important to fully understand each partner's perspective. Once again, Mahdiya stated that she thought it was morally wrong. She also had difficulty understanding Amir's desire to masturbate when he was married. Amir said that he was unsure why he felt the need to masturbate when he was married, but that he did not think it was wrong to do so. During the discussion, he looked at Mahdiya and said, "Would you rather I go find someone and actually cheat with them?" To which she stated, "You might as well, you're looking at lots of naked women anyways."

It became clear through this discussion that while there were religiously informed boundaries around the use of pornography, for both partners, the major issue with pornography was the way in which it impacted Mahdiya's self-esteem – knowing that her partner was turning toward pornography to meet his sexual needs instead of turning toward her. Additionally, it became clear that there was a lack of education about masturbation, the benefits of masturbation, and the role masturbation has in our sexual lives. Primarily, it was important for Mahdiya to understand that Amir's masturbatory habits could not be compared to the sexual interaction between them as a partner.

During the psychosexual education on both of these topics, it became clear that Amir was, in fact, avoiding sex with his partner. When I asked why, he stated that his wife made sex "too much work." Instead of being able to relax and enjoy himself, she had a number of things that he would have to do if he wanted to "get some" that night. When asked what he meant, he explained that the couple had seen a sex therapist after the birth of their first child. The therapist worked with Amir and Mahdiya to negotiate boundaries around sex. The previous therapist assumed that the couple could engage in more sex if Amir took on more responsibility in the household. In actuality, the couple was not engaging in sexual relations due to religious boundaries after childbirth and issues adjusting to being new parents. Nevertheless, the previous therapist's suggestions created a climate where Amir thought it was less work to simply masturbate than to engage intimately with his partner.

At this point in the therapeutic process, it was evident that they were underlying relational issues that created insecurity in the relationship and was responsible for the couple's sexual avoidance. I shared with the couple that I observed a pattern of sexual avoidance, going all the way back to the birth of their first child and being the cause and punishment of what was bringing them to therapy recently. This observation Mahdiya to weep. She stated that she had in fact begun avoiding sex after the birth of their first child because she felt insecure with her body. She also stated that her partners porn magnifies those insecurities, which is why she does not want to have sex until he stops looking at those images.

Amir was shocked at his partner's confession. He assured her that he was very attracted to her and that his porn usage did not replace her. It was then that he began to **incorporate his faith tradition** into the conversation, stating that he wanted to be with her intimately, but felt she was not interested, so he did not want to force her. This was the prime opportunity for me as the clinician to jump into the conversation. I asked the couples, "What do you think God wants from y'all's relationship? Do you think he wants y'all to be disconnected or find a way for the two of you to reconnect?" Both partners stated that God's will for their relationship was for them to have strong, emotional and sexual bonds and that they were willing to do whatever was necessary to reach that. This demonstrates one of the primary reasons that I enjoy working with religious couples – Their strong sense of commitment to their family.

Since both partners were on board to regain intimacy in their relationship, it was now time to **find creative solutions**. Since pornography was a presenting issue, and both partners felt that it was morally wrong, and was counter to their religious beliefs, I want to first start by addressing that issue. I recommend to Amir that whenever he feels like watching pornography, he would, instead, have a conversation with his wife. Simply having a conversation did not mean that they would have sex, nor did it mean that he would not watch pornography. It simply demonstrated to Mahdiya that she is his first choice and not the pornography. Since she had previously stated that she felt that Amir was replacing her with pornography and was affecting her self-esteem, this was done to help rebuild her self-confidence.

Another suggestion that was given to the couple was intimate play, instead of intercourse in situations where Mahdiya did not want to consent but also did not want to refuse her partner. In other words, when Amir would go to Mahdiya to express his sexual desire, if she did not feel like having sexual intercourse, the couple would find other ways to engage with each other intimately. This could include kissing while Amir masturbated or it could include Mahdiya pleasuring her partner manually or orally.

After three weeks of trying creative solutions, Amir expressed that he was no longer comfortable with using pornography due to his religious beliefs and asked for alternative suggestions.

While I initially suggested audio erotica or written erotic stories, he didn't seem comfortable with the former. However, he found reading erotic stories to be helpful in increasing his desire and fantasy towards his partner, which in turn excited Mahdiya. Upon discovering that Amir was fantasizing about her, Mahdiya decided to write several erotic stories as a playful birthday gift for her husband. This ignited passion and creativity in their relationship, and I suggested they begin to act out these fantasies in real life.

As the couple began to explore their fantasies, they discovered what each other enjoyed and added spontaneity and creativity to their love life. Over the course of five months, they reported having a regular sex life and feeling more connected to each other. Amir was no longer using pornography and was respecting his religious boundaries, although he still admitted to occasionally masturbating, which he enjoyed. Mahdiya stated that she finally enjoyed their sex life and had learned quite a bit about herself throughout the process. While there were still instances where she lacked self-confidence, she was able to recognize when her responses were based on her lack of self-esteem rather than her partner's behavior. Overall, the couple felt that they were having the best sex of their entire relationship.

Conclusion

All three Abrahamic faiths have boundaries around masturbation, with Christianity being the most liberally minded – depending on the denomination. Both Christianity and Islam encourage masturbation over sexual acts with another person with whom the person may not be married to. Judaism, on the other hand, holds an entirely different view. A competent sex therapist must understand these differences and be willing to explore the unique cognitive framework within each of these faith traditions concerning masturbation.

The three case studies in this chapter dealt with a very common issue that arises when working with religious patients. While most of the time, you will discover that the discussion around masturbation is connected to pornography usage, this is not always the case. However, when pornography is involved, all three Abrahamic faith traditions have strong boundaries against its usage. Therefore, it is helpful for clinicians to develop a list of alternatives to pornography usage that they can recommend to their patients. This topic will come up if working with religious persons for any length of time.

While it should go without saying, sex therapists should avoid recommending pornography usage when working with religious patients. This suggestion may seem obvious after reading the previous chapters but I cannot tell you the number of religious people who have told me that they left their previous therapist because they recommended something that was contrary to their morals. We should strive to be understanding and respectful, as demonstrated in the way that we present information, and in the solutions that we offer.

In none of the examples given in this chapter was the goal to change the patient's worldview concerning masturbation. Instead, the goal was to gain a greater understanding of their perspective as the clinician and help the patient to recognize their own sexual values. While in some cases, the patient abandons their religiously informed beliefs, this is also not the goal. Most importantly, is that the patient develops confidence in their sexual decision-making, regardless of what their faith tradition, society, or the clinician may say or think.

Notes

1 There are reports of clergy suggesting that individuals masturbate in order to avoid premarital sex or homosexual behavior. In these cases, masturbation has been described as the "lesser of two evils."

2 The aversion from using the term "addiction" does not indicate that the individual does not have a problem with pornography usage. They very well could have negative issues related to their use of such material. The distinction between out-of-control sexual behavior or compulsive sexual behavior and sexual or porn addiction should eventually be discussed with the religious patient. In the early stages of therapy, I suggest using the terminology that the patient uses when trying to understand, assess, and develop a treatment plan.

References

Alli, H. (2011). *Intimacy and the Sacred: In Muslim Communities*. iUniverse.

Hoagland, K. C., Rotruck, H. L., Moore, J. N., & Grubbs, J. B. (2023). Reasons for moral-based opposition to pornography in a US nationally representative sample. *Journal of Sex & Marital Therapy*. DOI: 10.1080/0092623X.2023.2186992

Lloyd, C. E.M. (2021). Contending with spiritual reductionism: Demons, shame, and dividualising experiences among Evangelical Christians with mental distress. *Journal of Religion and Health*, *60*(4), 2702–2727. DOI:10.1007/s10943-021-01268-9

Neves, S. (2021). The religious disguise in "sex addiction" therapy. *Sexual and Relationship Therapy*, *37*(3), 299–313. DOI: 10.1080/14681994.2021.2008344

Nie, F., & Olson, D. V.A. (2016). Demonic influence: The negative mental health effects on belief in demons. *Journal for the Scientific Study of Religion*, *55*(3), 498–515. DOI: 10.1111/jssr.12287

Patterson, R., & Price, J. (2012). Pornography, religion, and the happiness gap: Does pornography impact the actively religious differently? *Journal for the Scientific Study of Religion*, *51*(1), 79–89. DOI: 10.1111/j.1468–5906.2011.01630.x

Perry, S. L., & Whitehead, A. L. (2019). Only bad for believers? Religion, pornography use, and sexual satisfaction among American men. *The Journal of Sex Research*, *56*(1), 50–61. DOI: 10.1080/00224499.2017.1423017

Rassool, G. H., & Khan, M. A. (2020). *Sexuality Education from an Islamic Perspective*. Cambridge Scholars Publishing.

8

Premarital Sex

Introduction

Sex before marriage is a topic that often comes up when working with religious patients, regardless of whether they identify as Christian, Jewish, or Muslim. Across all three Abrahamic faith traditions, premarital sex is discouraged or even forbidden. For many religious individuals, the idea of abstaining from sex until marriage is an important part of their moral and spiritual values. However, in today's society, premarital sex has become more accepted and normalized. As a result, many religious patients may struggle with conflicting feelings and desires when it comes to their sexual behavior. They may feel pressure from their peers, partners, or even their own biological urges to engage in sexual activity before marriage, even if it goes against their religious teachings.

In addition to the physiological and biological factors that may lead a person to engage in sexual activity, various variables have been identified that are associated with a higher likelihood of premarital sex among religious individuals. According to Behulu et al. (2019), one of the leading reasons for premarital sex is the inability to discuss sex among peers. This lack of communication and knowledge-sharing can result in individuals making uninformed decisions regarding their sexual health and engaging in behaviors that may be against their religious beliefs.

DOI: 10.4324/9781003242017-12

Likewise, research has shown that the source of authority for religious individuals can also impact their likelihood of engaging in premarital sex. According to Uecker and Froese (2019), those who identify as religious individualists and rely on their own interpretation of God's will, rather than institutional sources of authority, such as the Bible or religious teachings, are more likely to engage in premarital sex. This may be due to the individualistic nature of their beliefs, which allows for more flexibility and subjective interpretation of religious principles.

This aligns with the findings of Brooks and Weitzman's (2022) research, which revealed an interesting irony in the relationship between religiosity and sexual behavior. According to their results, the more religious a young woman is, the less likely she is to engage in sexual activity and to use hormonal contraception in a given week. However, when they do engage in sexual activity and use a hormonal method, the more religious a young woman is, the more likely she is to use condoms. This finding could suggest that religious women who engage in sexual activity are more conscientious about preventing sexually transmitted infections (STIs) while still adhering to their religious beliefs regarding contraception.

Since premarital sex is a common cause of emotional and spiritual concern for many religious individuals, it will inevitably come up within sex therapy. Thus, gaining insight into effective interventions to assist religious individuals in addressing their concerns related to premarital sex can be beneficial. One approach that can be helpful when working with religious patients struggling with premarital sex is to explore the underlying beliefs and values that inform their decisions. Research indicates that even among those who have sex before marriage, their sexual ethics are still informed by their religious tradition (Huygens, 2022). We can help our patients to examine their own attitudes towards sex and relationships and to identify any conflicts or contradictions between their religious teachings and their personal desires. By fostering an open and non-judgmental dialogue, we can help our patients to gain a deeper understanding of their own motivations and values and to make more informed choices about their sexual behavior.

Therapist Bias Check

1. Am I being influenced by my own personal beliefs and values when working with a patient who associates sexual activity with morality and places importance on virginity and premarital sex?
2. Am I making assumptions about this patient's beliefs and values based on their religion or cultural background, and am I taking the time to understand their unique perspective and experiences?

Case Study 1 – Benjamin

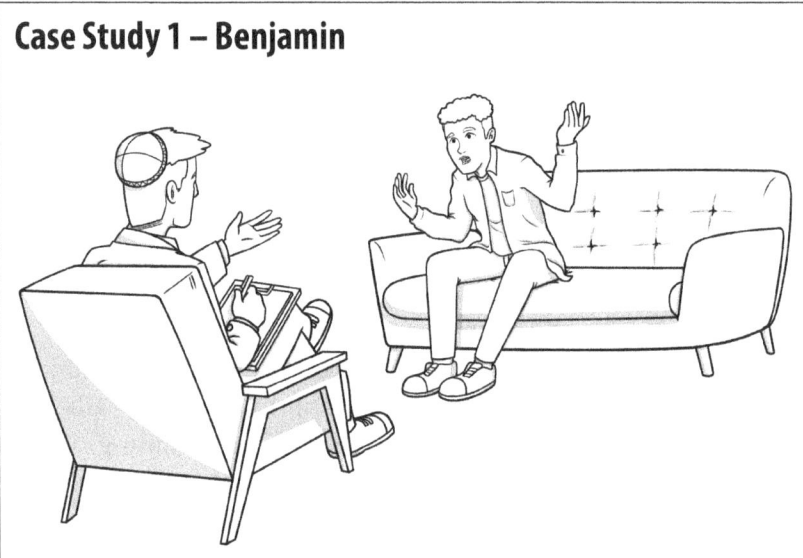

Benjamin, a 23-year-old Jewish male, has been struggling with his sexual orientation since he was 16 years old. He identifies as gay, but he also acknowledges that he might be bisexual. Growing up, Benjamin's family and the Reform community in which they belonged were very supportive of his sexual orientation. He recalls numerous conversations with the community rabbi about his sexuality but never remembers any discussion about safety.

During college, Benjamin found solace in a Jewish LGBTQ student program, where he felt a sense of belonging and felt like he was making a difference through activism and outreach. He found the environment to be very accepting of his sexual orientation, which he describes as encouraging. However, recently, Benjamin was diagnosed with a sexually transmitted infection, which left him feeling embarrassed, regretful, and humiliated.

Benjamin has been struggling with blaming his "sex-positive" religious community, which he believes encouraged his unsafe sexual behavior. He feels that the community or the rabbi should have discussed with him the importance of safe sex. This situation has left Benjamin feeling lost, alone, and questioning his faith in God. He has not yet told his parents about his STI status and feels like giving up on life.

Initial Interaction

When I first met Benjamin, he appeared nervous and hesitant to discuss his sexual interests, orientation, and recent STI diagnosis. As we began our session using the PLISSIT model, I asked for his permission to discuss these topics, recognizing that everyone has different levels of comfortability with sex. Benjamin agreed to the discussion, and I encouraged him to give himself permission to talk about sex as well. I acknowledged that talking about sex can sometimes seem taboo and uncomfortable, especially in the context of religion, and asked if he felt he could engage in the conversation. He responded with a nod.

Step 1 – Identify

Benjamin is experiencing feelings of guilt and shame as a result of his sexual behavior, which is compounded by the fact that he has contracted an STI. He is deeply embarrassed about the situation and is fearful that others will find out. However, he appears to have a misconception of sex positivity, believing it to mean that anything goes when it comes to sex, rather than a more nuanced approach that emphasizes consensual and ethical behavior. Furthermore, Benjamin has difficulty taking responsibility for his own actions and instead seeks to place blame on his religious community. This can be a significant barrier to making progress in therapy, as it is important for Benjamin to acknowledge his own agency and work towards making positive changes in his behavior.

Step 2 – Uncover

While it is true that most branches of Judaism have made strides in incorporating LGBTQ individuals into communal life, The Reform movement in Judaism is generally recognized as being more accepting and supportive of the LGBTQ community than other branches. his can be attributed to a number of factors, including their emphasis on social justice and inclusivity, as well as a general trend towards more progressive attitudes in areas such as gender and sexuality. These aspects can create a more welcoming and inclusive atmosphere for LGBTQ individuals seeking to connect with their faith. However, in Benjamin's case, his understanding of the Reform movement's acceptance of the LGBTQ community may be misguided. He may have confused the acceptance of LGBTQ individuals with an acceptance of any sexual behavior without boundaries or consequences.

Step 3 – Recognize

Due to my religious background, I had to be mindful of the potential for personal bias to impact my work with Benjamin. In this case, there was an inter-religious conflict as Benjamin came from a Reform tradition of Judaism, while I came from a more traditional Orthodox practice of Judaism. It was important for me to recognize the potential for my own beliefs and values to influence my interactions with Benjamin, particularly in discussions around sex and Judaism.

As we began our sessions, I made a conscious effort to remain open-minded and non-judgmental when Benjamin shared his beliefs and experiences around sexuality as it related to what he had been taught in his religious community. This involved listening actively and asking questions to gain a deeper understanding of his perspective, without imposing my own views on him. Despite our differing religious backgrounds, we were able to establish a respectful and collaborative relationship that allowed us to work together towards his goals.

I also recognized the importance of being knowledgeable about different sects within my own faith tradition and their teachings on sexuality, so that I could better understand Benjamin's perspective and provide appropriate guidance.

This involved doing research and seeking guidance from other professionals with expertise in inter-religious conflicts and sexual health.

Overall, navigating an inter-religious conflict in therapy requires a willingness to be open-minded, non-judgmental, and knowledgeable about different religious traditions. It also involves recognizing the potential for personal bias and taking steps to mitigate its impact on the therapeutic relationship.

Step 4 – Develop

As Benjamin's therapist, it was essential to provide a safe space for him to express his feelings, beliefs, and emotions without judgment. He already felt a sense of self-condemnation due to his sexual behavior. Since he was really having emotional difficulty over his recent STI diagnosis, it was also important to validate his experiences and empathize with his struggles. It was also very important to provide him with some **psychosexual education** that would partly destigmatize his recent diagnosis as well as help him to make healthier sexual health decisions in the future.

The psychosexual education given to Benjamin focused on safer sex practices. The discussion began about the use of the term *sexually transmitted infection* (STI) over the more traditional *sexually transmitted disease* (STD). It was explained to Benjamin that all diseases must have symptoms by definition, however, this is not the case with infections. This led to further discussion about the importance of regular testing so that infections can be spotted early on and, in most cases, can be treated. With all patients, I explain that the only safe sex is no sex, however, there are ways to reduce the risk and spread of sexually transmitted infections, such as using condoms (Davids et al., 2021).

There is no doubt that the stigma associated with sexually transmitted infections can make it difficult for people to seek testing and treatment (Sharma et al., 2022). Many individuals are afraid of being judged or ostracized for their sexual behavior or diagnosis. Moreover, there is a lack of information about how testing works and what the process entails, which can contribute to anxiety. To address this issue, several testing options were presented to Benjamin, including anonymous clinics and at-home testing kits. These options aim to reduce the stigma associated with testing, as individuals can test in a more private and comfortable setting. By normalizing the testing process, it was my goal to help Benjamin become more comfortable with the idea of being tested and receiving treatment in the future.

Several treatment options for STIs were also presented to Benjamin. This helped him recognize that his fear of being diagnosed with an STI was unfounded, as there are effective treatments available. Also, I wanted to destigmatize the notion of having an STI, as it is a common occurrence and does not reflect on an individual's character or morality. By providing this education and resources on testing and treatment options, I wanted Benjamin to be more informed and empowered to take control of his sexual health. Another important element that impacted him was his lack of willingness to take responsibility for his sexual behavior.

Benjamin's reaction to contracting an STI was to blame his reform Jewish community for their supposed lack of emphasis on safe sex practices. He believed that their accepting and sex-positive attitude had given him a false sense of security and led to his reckless behavior. However, this blame-shifting mentality is not uncommon among individuals who feel shame and guilt over their sexual behaviors. It was necessary for Benjamin to recognize that he is ultimately responsible for his own choices and actions and that blaming others is not a productive way to address his situation.

I recommend it to Benjamin, the following three steps to help him take responsibility for his own sexual health:

1. **Acknowledge the behavior:** The first step to taking responsibility is to acknowledge the behavior that led to poor sexual health decisions. It's important for an individual to be honest with themselves about the choices they made and how they may have contributed to the situation.
2. **Take action to address the situation:** Taking responsibility also involves taking action to address the situation.

This may include getting tested for STIs, seeking medical treatment, and discussing the situation with sexual partners. One should not put off such action due to guilt, shame, or inconvenience.

3. **Pre-plan your sexual decision-making:** Waiting until the moment can lead to impulsive and regretful decisions. Thus, one should plan and decide beforehand how they will approach a given situation. This can help to reduce the likelihood of negative outcomes and promote positive sexual health choices (Davids et al., 2021).

Next, I wanted to address Benjamin's need to reconnect with his religious community. I suggested **incorporating his faith tradition** into our therapy sessions. With Benjamin's consent, I reached out to his local rabbi to discuss some of the concerns that Benjamin had expressed about the messaging he received from the community. While I did not disclose Benjamin's sexual health status, I explained that he was struggling with feelings of guilt and shame and hoped to find a way to reconcile his faith with his sexuality. The rabbi was receptive to my request and agreed to participate in a joint session with Benjamin to provide a safe space for him to express his feelings and receive guidance on how to reconcile his beliefs with his sexual behavior. By incorporating his faith tradition into therapy, we were able to provide Benjamin with a holistic approach to healing that addressed both his spiritual and emotional needs.

Additionally, I wanted to incorporate his faith tradition and some **creative solutions** to help him move past his guilt and shame. Since I wanted to encourage him to focus on the present in the future, rather than dwelling in the past, I thought it could be useful to explore his relationship with God, and how his faith could support him and move forward from this challenging experience.

Over the four and a half months that I worked with Benjamin, he made significant strides in personal growth and self-discovery. Throughout our sessions, he was able to achieve a sense of coherence and consistency between his sexuality, including his previous mistakes, and his perception of the role his religious community has in his life and personal decision-making. He took ownership of his actions and developed valuable tools to help him make informed decisions about his sexual health in the future while staying true to himself. This progress allowed him to feel more empowered and confident in his life overall.

Case Study 2 – Amber

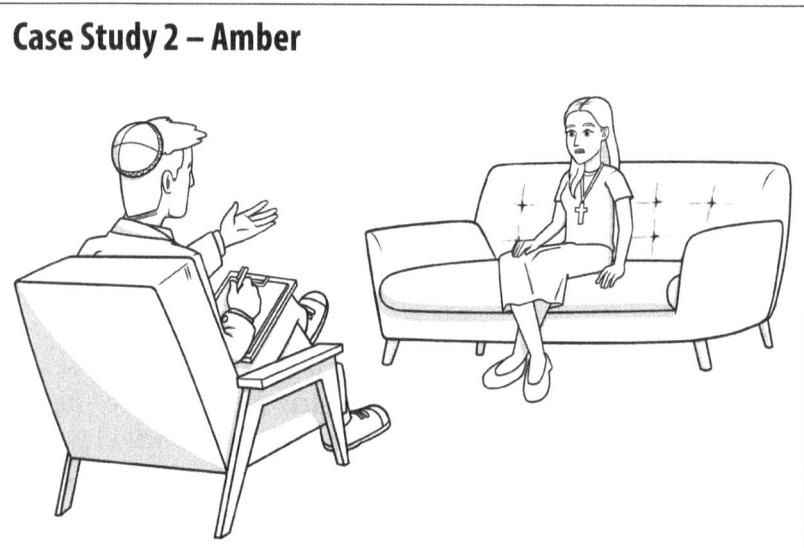

Amber is a 26-year-old woman who is actively involved in her nondenominational church. She devotes much of her time volunteering for the church, teaching Sunday School, and singing in the choir. She admits that she has been engaging in premarital sex, which goes against the teachings of her church, and this has led to considerable distress. This has caused Amber to struggle with severe anxiety and depression lately, primarily due to her fear of contracting an STI, getting pregnant unexpectedly, people in her church finding out about her sexual behavior, and going to hell. She is afraid that if anyone in her church, especially her pastor, finds out, she will be ostracized and shamed. Additionally, since she still lives with her parents, and fears that they will kick her out of the house if they find out.

Amber disclosed that she has been secretly bringing her partners into the Sunday School classroom where she teaches when the church is empty in order to engage in sexual activity with random partners that she finds online. This compounds her anxiety and intensifies her fear of eternal damnation. She feels guilty about her sexual desires and wants to be a good Christian, but the conflict between her faith and her sexuality has been causing her a lot of distress. Amber has sought therapy to help her reconcile her faith with her sexual desires and to receive support in managing her anxiety and depression.

Initial Interaction

After getting to know Amber during our sessions, it became clear that her strong involvement in the church had brought on a significant amount of anxiety and fear. She believed that her active involvement meant she was held to a higher level of accountability. During our sessions, Amber expressed her deep concern about her sexual behavior and how it could negatively impact her status within the church community. She explained that she had been engaging in sexual activity outside of marriage and was afraid of being judged or shamed if her behavior were to become known. Additionally, she explained that if anyone found out, it would mean that she would be relieved of her position within the church.

During our first session, when the PLISSIT model was introduced, Amber stated that she had no problems with us discussing sex or sexual issues, but that she feared that someone in her religious community would discover what she disclosed. After assuring Amber of complete confidentiality, I told her that I would never speak with anyone in her community unless she thought it was necessary and I had her permission. She was satisfied by these commitments and seemed relieved to have someone whom she could finally discuss these issues with. Numerous times she mentioned how she has never had anyone to talk to about sexual topics before.

Step 1 – Identify

In Amber's case, the problem was her internal conflict between her faith and her sexual desires, which were causing her severe anxiety and depression. She was struggling with the guilt and shame associated with engaging in premarital sex, and her fear of ostracism and judgment from her church community was compounding her distress. Additionally, her fear of contracting STIs, getting pregnant, and going to hell was adding to her anxiety.

Step 2 – Uncover

Amber was actively involved in a conservative nondenominational church, which is a type of Christian church that is not formally aligned with any specific denomination or association of churches. In this context, personal faith, the Bible, and individual spiritual experiences are often emphasized over adherence to specific doctrines or creeds. Due to her religious beliefs, Amber understood premarital sex to be forbidden in the biblical text and therefore considered it a major sin that could cause one to spend eternity in hell.

To add to the complexity of the situation, studies indicate that within religious communities that disapprove of premarital sexual activity, females tend to be held to a higher standard of morality as male sexual desires are more commonly tolerated and accepted (Eriksson et al., 2013; Hawkey et al., 2018). Thus, Amber's emotional turmoil was partly due to her gender. She felt as though she was not living up to the expectations of her family, her church, and her God.

In cases where there is a systemic interaction between multiple systems, it is important to gather more information about the patient's experiences, beliefs, and values related to their presenting problem. In Amber's case, the following questions were useful in exploring her experiences and beliefs:

♦ *Can you tell me more about your beliefs about sex and sexuality within your church?*
♦ *How do you feel about engaging in premarital sex, and what are your fears and concerns related to it?*
♦ *How do you feel about the conflict between your faith and your sexuality, and how has it affected your mental health?*
♦ *Can you describe your experiences with guilt and shame related to your sexual desires?*

- *How important is your involvement in your church to you, and how do you think your church community would respond if they found out about your sexual activity?*
- *Can you tell me more about your relationship with your parents and how you think they would respond if they found out about your sexual activity?*

By exploring these questions, it was possible to gain a better understanding of Amber's experiences and beliefs related to her sexuality and her faith. This understanding then informed the approach to treatment and helped develop interventions that are consistent with Amber's beliefs and values while also addressing her anxiety and depression.

Step 3 – Recognize

As a clinician, I noticed many aspects of this particular case that could indicate spiritual abuse. Primarily Amber's fear of what will happen to her if she is "found out" by members of her community or her pastor. It is important, however, not to project this assumption at the early stages of treatment as it is uncertain if Amber's fears are based upon actual events that have taken place within her community in the past, or if she is assuming these consequences based upon the way she has interpreted some of the messaging delivered concerning sexual behavior and norms. I would ask questions such as:

- *Has there ever been a situation in your church where the pastor found out someone was having premarital sex? Share with me what happened.*

The other aspect that could trigger a therapist's bias is the connection between sexual behavior and morality. A non-religious sex therapist could be offended by such a correlation, so it would be important to reflect on their own values and biases before engaging in therapy with a patient whose beliefs differ from their own. The therapist must strive to maintain a non-judgmental attitude and an open mind toward the patient's beliefs and values, regardless of their personal beliefs. It is crucial to provide a safe and supportive space for the patient to discuss their concerns without fear of judgment or shame. By recognizing and addressing their own biases, the therapist can ensure that they are providing effective and ethical treatment.

Step 4 – Develop

During our sessions, Amber and I worked to identify some of the negative self-talk and irrational fears that were contributing to her anxiety and depression, as recognized in Step 2. We found that much of her negative self-talk stemmed from her church's teachings, which suggests that Amber based her self-worth on sexual purity and controlling sexual urges. This is consistent with Gish's (2018) research findings. Furthermore, Amber's fears were consistent with the experiences of others who were involved in Christian communities with comparable beliefs, as demonstrated by Klein (2018).

Based on our understanding of the negative self-talk and irrational fears that were contributing to Amber's anxiety and depression, I developed strategies to help her move towards a healthier approach to her sexuality and relationships, while still honoring her religious beliefs. Creating a safe and non-judgmental environment for Amber was crucial for her to explore her thoughts and emotions, and I made sure to acknowledge the importance of her faith and values, as well as the role her family played in her life. This allowed her to feel at ease and open up to me, knowing that her beliefs would not be attacked. It also helped her feel safe in her disclosures knowing that others would have no way of knowing she was talking to me.

As part of our approach, I recommended that we start with **psychosexual education** to help Amber stay safe during her sexual encounters. Addressing Amber's fears and anxiety related to contracting STIs or unintended pregnancies was an essential measure. This importance was further magnified by Amber's disclosure that she lacked any form of sex education during her formative years, receiving no guidance from her parents or school. Research conducted by Zori et al. (2023) underscores the significance of such

education, highlighting that individuals who lack comprehensive sex education are more susceptible to unwanted
pregnancies and face a heightened risk of contracting STIs.
In this particular case, the limited information provided in
the psychosexual education part of treatment included the
following topics:

1. **STI prevention:** This could include information on how
   to use condoms and other barrier methods, as well as
   how to get tested for STIs and what to do if she were to
   receive a positive diagnosis.
2. **Pregnancy prevention:** This could include information
   on different forms of birth control and how they work, as
   well as how to access and use them effectively.
3. **Sexual pleasure and communication:** This could
   involve discussing how to communicate with sexual
   partners about likes and dislikes, boundaries, and consent, as well as exploring different ways to experience
   sexual pleasure.
4. **Healthy relationships:** This could involve exploring
   what makes a healthy relationship, including factors
   such as mutual respect, communication, and trust, as
   well as identifying warning signs of unhealthy or abusive relationships.
5. **Sex and spirituality:** This could involve exploring how
   spirituality and sexuality intersect, and how Amber can
   integrate her religious beliefs into her sexual experiences
   in a way that feels comfortable and authentic for her.

We also **incorporated her faith tradition** into our work. I did
this by taking a text from the New Testament that she frequently
quoted as the foundation of her belief that premarital sex was
immoral and wrong:

Flee from sexual immorality. Every other sin a person
commits is outside the body, but the sexually immoral
person sins against his own body.

1 Corinthians 6:18 (*English Standard Version*)

I then had her continue with the next two verses of the texts, which state:

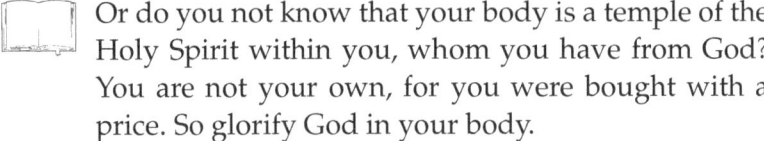 Or do you not know that your body is a temple of the Holy Spirit within you, whom you have from God? You are not your own, for you were bought with a price. So glorify God in your body.
          1 Corinthians 6:19–20 (*English Standard Version*)

These texts allow for the conversation to be shifted toward the idea of her body being a "temple." This then led to a series of questions intended to cause Amber to establish her own understanding of the text and determine if it is different than that of her churches or not.

◆   *What does it mean that your body is a temple of God?*

"It means that I am God's temple and that he dwells in me."

◆   *So God created you, and he dwells in you?*

"Yes, exactly."

◆   *What exactly does that mean? Like what are the implications?*

"It means that I need to be careful what I do because God is inside of me."

◆   *You wouldn't possibly think that God is going to hell right?*

"Of course not, that's not a thing."

◆   *Well, I say that because, if God is dwelling in you, even if we look past the fact that – and I think you would agree – that God is too magnetic and unfathomable to dwell exclusively inside of one person, if you go hell and God is dwelling in you, that would seem as though God would also be going to hell.*

"Well no, God isn't going to hell, it's more like we need to be mindful of what we do since God dwells inside of us."

♦ *Ah, I see, so it is more of a metaphor.*

"Yeah, sort of. It is like a reality that God is inside of us when we receive the Holy Spirit but it is also symbolic."

♦ *What does the metaphoric part mean? Like what are the application?*

"That we need to be aware of how we treat our bodies and to treat them with respect and honor since they are God's Temple."

♦ *I see, so it is important that we are mindful of the things we do in relation to our bodies.*

"Yes."

♦ *And in doing that, would you say that we are honoring God?*

"Absolutely."

This conversation allowed me to shift the focus on honoring God instead of her fear of going to hell. Therefore, instead of framing it like the text does, where the focus was on "sin," I shifted the focus to other parts of the text, which focus on honoring God. This was a positive move in helping Amber gain autonomy over her sexual behavior. For homework, I asked her to come up with a list of ways she could honor God with her body.

In actuality, I was not too concerned with what Amber would put on her list. The aim was to get her to start being mindful of how she was honoring her body – and thus, honoring the "temple of God" according to her theological perspective. This became part of the **creative solutions** to help her reconcile her religious beliefs with her sexual behavior. After sharing her list, I asked her if there were ways she could honor her body when engaging in sex. She stated that it would be important to keep her body healthy and not to be exposed to STIs.

Together, we explored ways for her to respect her body by using safer sex practices, such as using condoms or birth control. We likewise discussed the way in which she found her partners. During this discussion, Amber disclosed that she met up with random men in order to feel desired and wanted. She then disclosed that while she would like to have a committed relationship, she doesn't think that she is good enough for a partner and that no one would want to be with her, especially if they found out she has been having sex. In this moment, it became apparent that the mechanism that she was using to deal with her low self-esteem was just complicating the issue even further. Therefore, I found it imperative to help Amber set her own healthy boundaries around sex, which took into account her religious convictions and the way in which she felt about herself.

Amber made a personal decision to abstain from engaging in sexual activities with multiple partners and instead committed herself to only being sexually active within committed relationships. She also recognized the importance of using contraception during these encounters. While these boundaries alleviated her spiritual anxiety, she still harbored concerns about the potential consequences if her parents or someone from her church were to discover her sexual activity.

To address this, I introduced Amber to the concept of limited disclosure. Research, as highlighted by Gyan (2018), suggests that females who are sexually active in religious communities often choose to keep their relationships secret as a strategic approach to avoid ostracization. With this in mind, I recommended that Amber refrain from disclosing this information to individuals within her religious community or those who have connections to her family. Amber agreed that this approach would be wise and decided to follow it.

Furthermore, Amber also made the resolution to no longer engage in sexual behavior within the church's Sunday School classrooms. She saw this as a source of her spiritual anxiety. We discussed how such behavior was not being authentic to herself as it was not respectful to her religious beliefs, community, or the children that she taught each week. She also stated that this was one of the biggest reasons why she felt that she would eventually get caught. Later she disclosed that by implementing this simple boundary, she had a significant reduction in her anxiety and fear of hell.

In the following weeks, I provided unwavering support to Amber as she embarked on the journey of integrating these boundaries into her life and asserting autonomy over her own sexuality for the first time. No longer driven by the need for external validation or shackled by the fear of eternal consequences, Amber now made well-informed decisions that resonated with her inner truth.

As our sessions progressed, it became evident that her confidence had significantly grown since our initial meeting. Amber was steadily moving towards self-actualization, embracing an authentic way of living that aligned with her values and desires. She skillfully reconciled her religious beliefs with her evolving sexual behavior, allowing herself to lead a more fulfilling life. Amber's path toward personal fulfillment and harmony exemplified the remarkable progress she had achieved.

Case Study 3 – Khalid and Fatima

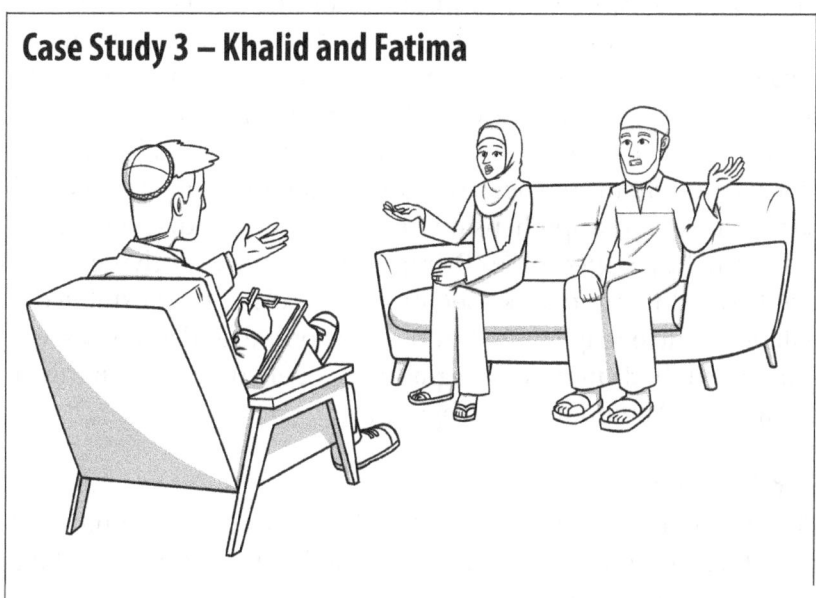

Khalid, 21, and Fatima, 19, were both raised in Muslim households with strict adherence to religious traditions and values. Their families arranged for them to meet, and after a brief courtship, they decided to get married. Although they were young, they were excited to start their life together as a married couple.

On their wedding night, Khalid was shocked when he did not see any blood on the bedsheets after they had sex for the first time. In his culture and religion, it is expected that a woman will bleed on her wedding night as a sign of her virginity. Khalid immediately assumed that Fatima was not a virgin before their marriage, which is a significant issue in their culture and religion.

Khalid believes that Fatima deceived him by not telling him that she was not a virgin, and he wants to annul the marriage according to Muslim law. Fatima, on the other hand, maintains that she is a virgin and is deeply hurt by Khalid's accusations. She is confused and frustrated by the situation, as she has no way of proving her innocence to Khalid.

Initial Interaction

Considering the age of the patients and the delicate nature of their situation, I promptly introduced the PLISSIT model and explicitly sought their permission to engage in discussions pertaining to sexual matters. This step held exceptional significance, given the sensitive context of this case. Both partners willingly granted me permission, extending it not only to themselves but also to each other. Throughout the therapy session, their demeanor suggested nervousness and apprehension, reflective of their discomfort not only with the prospect of sex therapy but also the underlying issues that had led them to seek therapy. Nonetheless, they exhibited a willingness to engage with the questions posed, and as the session progressed, both individuals gradually opened up, sharing their thoughts and emotions more openly.

Step 1 – Identify

The presenting issue was Khalid's misunderstanding and misinformed view of virginity, which led him to assume that his partner was not a virgin on their wedding night.

Step 2 – Uncover

In this instance, the underlying issue is the same as the presenting problem. Khalid believes that Fatima is not a virgin due to the fact that there were no traces of blood after they had sex for the first time. This belief demonstrates faulty cognition on the part of Khalid as the Quran does not state such, however, the practice has been adopted within certain segments of the Islamic tradition, most likely due to Western influence. However, Islamic law does allow for a man to get a divorce or annul the wedding if he discovers that his wife was not a virgin.

In this instance, the underlying religious issue is identical to the initial presenting problem. Khalid is of the belief that Fatima is not a virgin, as he did not observe any blood during their first sexual encounter. While Khalid's conviction reflects flawed reasoning, as the Quran does not explicitly state that the presence of blood is a sign of virginity, this practice has been adopted by certain segments of the Islamic tradition, potentially as a result of Western influence. In fact, the bride could be rejected by her husband, the marriage could be annulled, and she could be ostracized by her family and community, according to Chyssides et al. (2013, 40).

Step 3 – Recognize

When dealing with cases related to virginity, a sex-positive therapist may hold certain biases and prejudices in response to a patient's faulty cognitive constructs concerning virginity that reinforce harmful patriarchal notions that stigmatize women. These biases could potentially lead to the stigmatization of women who are not virgins. In such cases, it is essential for the therapist to recognize and acknowledge any biases they may have and take steps to avoid crossing professional boundaries that could be detrimental to their Muslim patient.

If a therapist is experiencing bias, they should consult with a clinical supervisor and a religious advisor to ensure that they are not imposing their personal beliefs onto the therapy sessions. It is crucial for the therapist to maintain a professional and ethical demeanor to ensure that their patient's needs and goals are being prioritized. By seeking guidance and advice from qualified professionals, the therapist can ensure that they are providing appropriate and culturally sensitive therapy to their Muslim patients.

Step 4 – Develop

When the couple agreed to attend therapy together, I noticed that Khalid was demonstrating a willingness to work on his marriage and was open to hearing what Fatima had to say, despite the strong feelings of anger and disappointment he was experiencing. He had many thoughts and emotions to share, feeling that Fatima had misled and betrayed him. In contrast, Fatima appeared to be withdrawn and hesitant to speak up during the session. From my assessment, I determined that her reluctance was likely due to the uncertainty and anxiety she was experiencing about her future, given the assumptions Khalid had made about her.

As a clinician, I always begin by asking for the patient's Permission to discuss sexual issues and ask specific questions related to their sexual concerns. In Fatima's case, she appeared to be closed off and uncomfortable discussing her issues. However, by taking this initial step, I was able to help her feel more at ease with the therapeutic process and give herself permission to discuss topics that she may not have felt comfortable discussing before. This approach allowed us to establish a foundation of trust and respect, which was crucial in helping her feel more comfortable opening up and exploring her concerns.

My treatment plan began with **psychosexual education**. In this instance, I believed that the education would help Khalid discover his misunderstanding concerning virginity as well as help Fatima feel less anxious and open up in the therapy room. The focus on the sex education was on the social construct of virginity and the false notion that virginity status can be determined by examination. I began by explaining that the hymen is not a seal that closes the entrance to the vagina and that some women are even born without hymens (Nagoski, 2015, 27–29).

Additionally, it was explained that the condition of the hymen is not an indication of virginity, citing research which noticed that some sex workers still had intact hymens (Dhall, 1995).

This information seemed to be surprising to both partners. Khalid raised a question about why some women bleed during sex, and I took the opportunity to explain that bleeding occurs because of vaginal tearing. I went on to explain that vaginal tearing can happen for a number of reasons, including the stretching of the vaginal canal during intercourse, lack of lubrication, or when sex is particularly rough. This information seemed to satisfy Khalid's curiosity and allowed us to have a more open and honest discussion about sexual health and anatomy.

This opened the door to discussing with the couple the dangers associated with holding rigid beliefs about virginity, particularly when these beliefs are founded on false assumptions. I shared with them some of the devastating consequences that many women face in countries where virginity testing is still practiced (Hegazy & Al-Rukban, 2012). For example, victims of sexual violence may not be believed when they come forward with their stories, or they may be subjected to a loss of dignity and respect by both authorities and family members.

At this point in the therapeutic process, Khalid accepted the fact that Fatima may not have been lying to him, and he apologized to her for his accusations against her. This led to the **incorporation of their faith tradition** into the treatment in order to bring healing in the relationship and strengthen their bond (Olson et al., 2015). Collectively we discussed the importance of marriage in Islam and the supporting role of husband and wife within that marital bond. Khalid expressed his commitment toward his partner and once again asked her forgiveness for the way he previously acted. Fatima finally opened up and told Khalid how much his accusations against her hurt her but that she forgave him and wanted to move forward.

In this particular case, there was no need to **find creative solutions** since the major issue revolved around a lack of understanding. Fortunately, providing Limited Information and Specific Suggestions was all that was needed. As a clinician, it was a deeply satisfying experience to witness the transformation of the couple's relationship dynamics. Through therapy, they were able to learn effective communication skills that allowed them to express their feelings openly and honestly. This newfound ability to communicate effectively helped them understand each other's perspective and led to a deepening of their emotional connection. It was gratifying to see how this communication led to displays of vulnerability in the form of apologies and forgiveness, demonstrating a willingness to let go of the past and move towards a brighter future together

Conclusion

Premarital sex is a common issue among religious patients of all three Abrahamic faith traditions, but the way in which it impacts a person's daily and spiritual life can differ greatly, as shown in the three case studies presented in this chapter. As a clinician, it is crucial to understand how complicated this topic can be and how challenging it can be for individuals to navigate.

Moreover, there are other common ways in which sexual behavior before marriage could be present when working with religious patients. These may include patients feeling guilty or ashamed, struggling with their own moral beliefs and values, or experiencing conflicts with their religious communities – especially in terms of feeling afraid of being caught or their sexual behavior becoming known by members of their religious community and particularly clergy.

In addition, patients may have misconceptions or faulty beliefs regarding the concept of virginity and the possibility of engaging in alternative sexual practices that they consider as an alternative to vaginal penetration. These frequently include:

1. Anal penetration instead of vagina penetration: Some religious patients may have the belief that they can maintain their virginity if they engage in anal sex instead of vaginal sex (Morhason-Bello et al., 2023). However, this can lead to unhealthy sexual practices as there is often a lack of education within their communities regarding safe anal sex and thus a higher prevalence of sexually transmitted infections (Calas et al., 2021).

2. Oral sex in the place of penetrative sex: Many religious patients hold the belief that oral sex is not considered sex, and thus may view it as a more acceptable alternative to penetrative sex. However, it is important to note that many of these individuals may not be aware of the risk of STIs that can be transmitted through oral sex, such as chlamydia, gonorrhea, syphilis, and herpes to name a few (Ballini et al., 2012; da Cunha et al., 2021).

3. Same sex interaction: It's an interesting paradigm to recognize that within some of the more conservative sects of these faith traditions, which hold strong beliefs against same-sex relationships often have individuals who had their first sexual encounters with someone of the same biological sex. This can be due to various reasons, such as (a) the belief that it does not count as a sexual encounter because it is with someone of the same sex, and (b) the increased likelihood of being alone with someone of the same sex.

By being aware of these variables, clinicians can better assess and notice factors that may not be as transparent upon a cursory glance of the case. At any rate, understanding these variables will help to provide the patient with the psychosexual education that they are lacking which can empower them to take autonomy over their sexual functioning and sexual health. As illustrated by the case studies presented in this chapter, guiding patients towards new perspectives without challenging their religious convictions, as it plays a crucial role in resolving their conflicts.

As therapists working with religious individuals, it's important to approach the topic of premarital sex with sensitivity and respect. We need to acknowledge the challenges and conflicts that our patients may be facing, while also being mindful of our own biases and beliefs. It's not our role to judge or impose our own values on our patients, but rather to support them in exploring their own beliefs and values and making their own decisions about their sexual behavior.

References

Ballini, A., Cantore, S., Fatone, L., Montenegro, V., De Vito, D., Pettini, F., Crincoli, V., Antelmi, A., Romita, P., Rapone, B., Miniello, G., Perillo, L., Grassi, F. R., & Foti, C. (2012). Transmission of nonviral sexually transmitted infections and oral sex. *Journal of Sexual Medicine*, *9*(2), 372–384. DOI: 10.1111/j.1743–6109.2011.02515.x

Behulu, G. K., Anteneh, K. T., & Aynalem, G. L. (2019). Premarital sexual intercourse and associated factors among adolescent students in Debre-Markos town secondary and preparatory schools, north west Ethiopia, 2017. *BMC Research Notes*, *12*(1), 95. DOI: 10.1186/s13104-019-4132-4

Brooks, I.H. M., & Weitzman, A. (2022). Religiosity and young unmarried women's sexual and contraceptive behavior: New evidence from a longitudinal panel of young adult women. *Demography*, *59*(3), 895–920. DOI: 10.1215/00703370–9931820

Calas, A., Zemali, N., Camuset, G., Jaubert, J., Manaquin, R., Saint-Pastou, C., Koumar, Y., Poubeau, P., Gerardin, P., & Bertolotti, A. (2021). Prevalence of urogenital, anal, and pharyngeal infections with chlamydia trachomatis, neisseria gonorrhoeae, and mycoplasma genitalium: A cross-sectional study in Reunion Island. *BMC Infectious Diseases*, *21*(1). DOI: 10.1186/s12879-021-05801-9

Chryssides, G. D., El Alami, D. S., & Cohn-Sherbok, D. (2013). *Love, Sex and Marriage: Insights from Judaism, Christianity and Islam*. SCM Press.

da Cunha, A. R., Bessel, M., Hugo, F. N., de Souza, F. M. A., Pereira, G. F. M., & Wendland, E. M. D. R. (2021). Sexual behavior and its association with persistent oral lesions: Analysis of the POP-Brazil Study. *Clinical Oral Investigations*, *25*(3), 1107–1116. DOI: 10.1007/s00784-020-03407-0

Davids, E. L., Y. Zembe, de Vries, P. J., Mathews, C., & Swatz, A. (2021). Exploring condom use decision-making among adolescents: the synergistic role of affective and rational processes. *BMC Public Health*, *21*(1). DOI: 10.1186/s12889–021–11926-y

Dhall, A. (1995). Adolescence: myths and misconceptions. *Health Millions*, *21*(3), 35–38.

Eriksson, E., Lindmark, G., Axemo, P., Haddad, B., & Ahlberg, B. M. (2013). Faith, premarital sex and relationships: Are church messages in accordance with the perceived realities of the youth? A qualitative study in KwaZulu-Natal, South Africa. *Journal of Religion and Health,* *52*(2), 454–466. DOI: 10.1007/s10943-011-9491-7

Gish, E. (2018). "Are you a 'trashable' Styrofoam cup?": Harm and damage rhetoric in the contemporary American sexual purity movement. *Journal of Feminist Studies in Religion, 34*(2), 5–22. DOI: 10.2979/ jfemistudreli.34.2.03

Gyan, S. E. (2018). Passing as "normal": Adolescent girls' strategies for escaping stigma of premarital sex and childbearing in Ghana. *SAGE Open, 8*(3). DOI: 10.1177/2158244018801421

Hawkey, A. J., Ussher, J. M., & Perz, J. (2018). Regulation and resistance: Negotiation of premarital sexuality in the context of migrant and refugee women. *The Journal of Sex Research, 55*(9), 1116–1133. DOI: 10.1080/00224499.2017.1336745

Hegazy, A. A., & Al-Rukban, M. O. (2012). Hymen: Facts and conceptions. *The Health, 3*(4), 109–115.

Huygens, E. (2022). "My dream is that I share the bed with only one man": Perceptions and practices of premarital sex among Catholic women in Belgium. *Social Compass, 69*(1), 59–75. DOI: 10.1177/00377686211049676

Klein, L. K. (2018). *Pure: Inside the Evangelical Movement That Shamed a Generation of Young Women and How I Broke Free.* Atria Books.

Morhason-Bello, I. O., Mitchell, K., Jegede, A. S., Adewole, I. F., Francis, S. C., & Watson-Jones, D. (2023). Heterosexual oral and anal sex: Perceptions, terminologies, and attitudes of younger and older adults in Ibadan, Nigeria. *Archives of Sexual Behavior, 52*(1), 161–175. DOI: 10.1007/s10508-022-02313-8

Nagoski, E. (2015). *Come as You Are: The Surprising New Science that Will Transform Your Sex Life.* Simon & Schuster.

Olson, J. R., Marshall, J. P., Goddard, H. W., & Schramm, D. G. (2015). Shared religious beliefs, prayer, and forgiveness as predictors of marital satisfaction. *Family Relations, 64*(5), 519–533. DOI: 10.1111/fare.12129

Sharma, B. B., Small, E., & Nikolova, S. P. (2022). Determinants of STI/HIV stigma and communication management among heterosexual couples in Kenya. *Journal of Applied Communication Research, 50*(2), 208–226. DOI: 10.1080/00909882.2021.1979240

Uecker, J. E., & Froese, P. (2019). Religious individualism and moral progressivism: How source of religious authority is related to attitudes about abortion, same-sex marriage, divorce, and premarital sex. *Politics and Religion*, *12*(2), 283–316. DOI: 10.1017/S1755048318000792

Zori, G., Waller, A. F., King, L., Duncan, R. P., Dayton, K., & Foti, S. (2023). The impact of state policy on adverse teen sexual health outcomes in the United States: A Scoping Review. *Sexuality Research and Social Policy*, *20*, 160–176. DOI: 10.1007/s13178-022-00770-3

9

Unconsummated Marriages

Introduction

In the current era, sex therapists are actively working towards broadening the definition of sex, recognizing that it encompasses more than just penis/vagina intercourse. Consequently, the concept of unconsummated marriages (UCM) may appear outdated or archaic. However, it remains a prevalent issue, particularly within religious and culturally conservative communities (Alla, 2017). It is not unheard of that a religious leader will recommend to a couple who has been unable to consummate their marriage to speak with a sex therapist to help resolve the issue. In fact, among those who work specifically with religious couples, this can be expected.

Unconsummated marriages typically arise from a variety of factors, including a lack of sufficient sexual information, sexual performance anxiety, limited privacy, a history of sexual abuse, unfounded fears, cultural and social influences, strict religious rules, societal and familial restrictions, and specific expectations regarding the first sexual intercourse (Bokaie et al., 2017). Vaginismus and dyspareunia are the number one female factor associated with unconsummated marriages (Xi et al., 2023). Premature ejaculation and erectile dysfunction are also frequently cited factors contributing to unconsummated marriages, affecting men's ability to achieve or sustain an erection (Mohamed Mohamed et al., 2021; Kojo et al., 2022; Xi et al., 2023).

DOI: 10.4324/9781003242017-13

Unconsummated marriages have a range of consequences for individuals and couples. These consequences may include feelings of guilt, shame, and inadequacy, diminished self-esteem, increased aggression, frustration, marital instability, potential infertility, and a higher likelihood of divorce (Bokaie et al., 2017). For the individual experiencing the sexual dysfunction, they have an overwhelming sense that something is wrong with them. They question why they are not able to engage in sexual intimacy with someone they love and care about. They feel guilty for not being able to open up to their partner. The partners also struggle with feelings of rejection and often blame themselves.

Acknowledging the significant influence of cultural factors on the occurrence and consequences of unconsummated marriages is crucial (Hosseini et al., 2017). Cultural norms, expectations, and beliefs pertaining to sex and marriage can create additional pressures and limitations for individuals, thereby further complicating the situation. It is not uncommon for patients to express their inability to perform sexually due to the overwhelming pressure imposed upon them. The transition from avoiding any form of sexual interaction to suddenly engaging in intercourse with a partner can be challenging. In many cases, these individuals may have never even shared a kiss with their partner before their wedding day, and yet now they are also expected to engage in intercourse with them.

The weight of these cultural and religious expectations, which often emphasize virginity and purity, can cause immense anxiety and difficulty in navigating intimate encounters. Such individuals may struggle with the expectations placed upon them and find it challenging to establish a comfortable and fulfilling sexual relationship. The fear of judgment, societal stigma, and the potential consequences of deviating from these expectations can further hinder their ability to explore their sexuality and experience sexual satisfaction within the confines of their cultural and religious beliefs. Thus, addressing unconsummated marriages is as complex as any other sexual issue that may arise in clinical practice.

Addressing unconsummated marriages requires a comprehensive approach that considers the physical, psychological, religious, and cultural aspects involved. Providing accurate sexual education, promoting open communication, addressing under-lying psychological factors, offering therapy and support, and challenging restrictive cultural and religious beliefs can all contribute to helping individuals and couples navigate and potentially overcome the challenges associated with unconsummated marriages.

Therapist Bias Check

1. Is my personal understanding of sexual activity potentially diminishing the distress experienced by the patient who is struggling with an unconsummated marriage?
2. Am I applying a one-size-fits-all approach to this situation, or am I considering the unique cultural, religious, and psychological factors that may be contributing to the unconsummated marriage?

Case Study 1 – David and Rivka

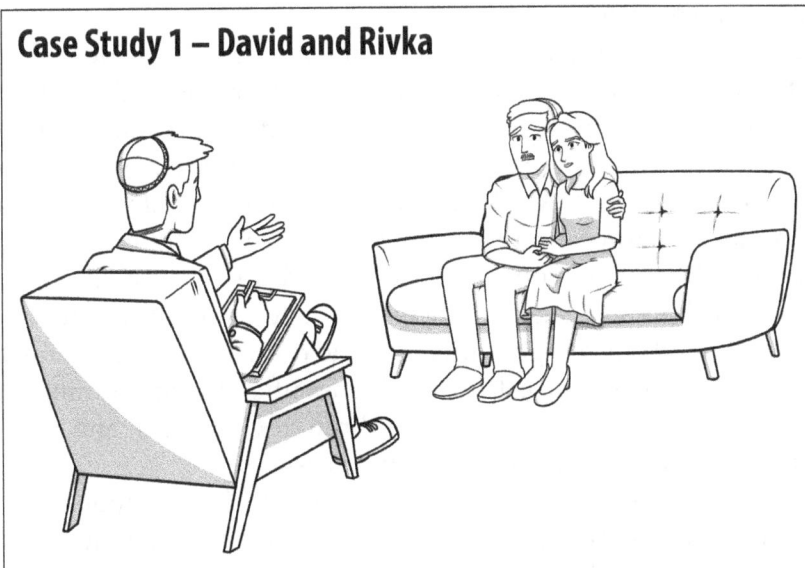

David, 24, and Rivka, 23, have been married for nine months but have not been able to have successful intercourse. Every time they try to get intimate, David ejaculates before he can even enter his partner. The couple are Orthodox Jews and hold the belief that sexual relations should only happen within the context of marriage and ejaculation should only take place within the vagina. David's inability to perform sexually is causing him great shame and guilt, and Rivka feels helpless because she cannot do anything to help him.

The couple rarely discusses the issue and neither understand why they are experiencing this problem. They are too embarrassed to speak with their parents or friends about it, and the situation has led them to the point of considering giving up on sex altogether. The couple's religious beliefs are adding to the pressure and shame they feel about their situation, and they do not know where to turn for help. They are both feeling distressed and frustrated, and the issue is starting to impact other aspects of their marriage. After speaking with their rabbi, they come to therapy with help to resolve the issue hoping to finally consummate their marriage.

Initial Interaction

Upon initial assessment of the couple, it became evident that David and Rivka shared a profound love for each other. Their strong devotion to their faith was also readily apparent, despite the additional emotional strain it imposed on their unconsummated marriage. Nevertheless, their religious beliefs served as a motivating force, propelling them to seek a resolution for their sexual difficulties. Both individuals held a deep reverence for family values and eagerly anticipated building a future together. Consequently, leveraging this intrinsic desire to create a family became a pivotal aspect of the therapeutic alliance, aiming to empower the couple to navigate through challenges and transcend feelings of frustration and helplessness.

As we began the assessment, the PLISSIT model was introduced, and I asked them for permission to speak about sexual issues. They quickly agreed to this, however, when I asked them to give themselves permission to discuss sexual topics, they were a bit more hesitant. For some, it may be easier to hear about these topics from a clinical professional, yet realizing that they have to be actively a part of the discussion is not in full consciousness.

This is the primary reason why PLISSIT is so effective in working with religious patients.

Step 1 – Identify

The couple presented with the issue of an unconsummated marriage caused by early ejaculation. This led to distress on the part of both partners. The husband felt he was failing by not being able to fulfill his duty as a husband and perform sexually, whereas the wife felt she was unable to help her partner. These additional emotional stressors only exacerbated the primary issue, which resulted in the couple deciding not to attempt any sexual interaction until they were able to find a solution.

Step 2 – Uncover

It could be easily overlooked that the couple's religious tradition contributes to their unconsummated marriage. The clinician should recognize this facet before automatically aiming to treat early ejaculation. Research suggests the commonality of unconsummated marriages among young Orthodox couples decreases the likelihood that the issue is linked to medical issues. Instead, it is most likely connected with emotional or dynamic factors (Ribner & Rosenbaum, 2005). Further research indicates that early ejaculation is the most common male sexual issue connected with unconsummated marriage (Friedman, 2019).

If early ejaculation does prove to be the cause of the unconsummated marriage, practitioners should be cautious about suggesting things that fall outside of the patient's religious belief system, such as masturbation. Additionally, it is important to note that while the male may be experiencing sexual dysfunction, the female partner may have overwhelming feelings of anxiety and guilt. As Ribner and Rosenbaum (2005) rightfully point out, "Religious restrictions on alternative sexual activities, such as mutual masturbation and oral sex, in Orthodox Jewish communities, may lead to the female partner feeling responsible for controlling her husband's orgasm, which can impact their sexual intimacy." From professional experience, it is not uncommon for this high level of anxiety on the part of the female to be a contributing factor to the development of some form of female genital pelvic pain/penetration disorder.

Step 3 – Recognize

Some practitioners could be confronted with bias associated with religious boundaries around masturbation. Nevertheless, despite the clinician's personal feelings, this situation should be a moment of creativity, where the therapist could find unique ways to overcome early ejaculation, and in this case, unconsummated marriages, within the framework of the patient's religiously informed boundaries. This is also an excellent opportunity for professional collaboration with the patient's religious leader. In many cases, it is already common for a rabbi to refer a community member to a sex therapist to resolve such an issue (Friedman, 2019). This shows the willingness of religious leaders to be involved in helping couples find solutions and improve their sexual connection.

Step 4 – Develop

According to current research, it is recommended to provide individualized treatment for couples diagnosed with unconsummated marriages. In the case of David and Rivka, the initial assessment and several early sessions were conducted within the context of couples therapy. This was a crucial period for gaining a comprehensive understanding of the various symptoms associated with their unconsummated marriage. Numerous studies have identified premature ejaculation as the primary cause of unconsummated marriages (Zargooshi, 2008; Alla, 2017), which was indeed the case with this particular couple. Within the first three sessions, Rivka expressed her fear that they would never be able to engage in sexual intercourse and shared her feelings of rejection stemming from the situation. These emotions are commonly experienced by couples facing unconsummated marriages (Ribner & Rosenbaum, 2005).

After gaining a thorough understanding of the situation, the couple received **psychosexual education** as part of their therapy. It was revealed that both David and Rivka had received no prior sex education before their marriage. The objective of psychosexual education was twofold: first, to provide them with basic information about their bodies and sexual functioning, and second, to alleviate some of the anxiety and emotions they were experiencing. By understanding the potential causes of early ejaculation, it was hoped that their feelings of fear, guilt, inadequacy, and rejection would diminish to some extent. The educational sessions were conducted individually with each partner, creating a space where they felt more comfortable discussing their limited knowledge and addressing any curiosities they had. This particular couple demonstrated an exceptional interest in human sexuality, leading to multiple sessions dedicated to psychosexual education. As therapy progressed, additional questions arose intermittently and were addressed accordingly.

Although both partners identified as frum (devoutly religious), David began expressing anger towards his faith tradition. He believed that his sexual dysfunction was caused by his religious background and felt frustrated that his religion had not prepared him for something that should come "naturally." It was evident from his expression that making such a statement was emotionally difficult for him. In an attempt to alleviate his distress, I emphasized that he should not harbor hostility towards his deeply meaningful religious beliefs. I explained that while sex is indeed a natural aspect of life (using the same terminology he had used previously), so is eating. However, just as you wouldn't expect a newborn to eat cholent (a popular Jewish dish typically consumed on Shabbat, especially within Ashkenazi communities), as someone who had never engaged in sexual activity before, this was his time to learn and explore. It was crucial to emphasize that he did not have to be perfect or get everything right on the first try, as everything was new to him. By relieving some of the self-imposed expectations, we were able to address the performance anxiety that significantly contributed to his early ejaculation.

Regarding Rivkah, it was crucial to alleviate her feelings of guilt and the belief that she was responsible for her husband's sexual issues. Over the course of two sessions, I worked with her to help her understand that she was not at fault and held no blame or responsibility in any way. Additionally, I began **incorporating**

her faith tradition into the therapeutic process, considering the emphasis placed on health, well-being, and life within Judaism. I framed the situation as an anatomical issue with a biological origin. Furthermore, I introduced the concept of marriage as a partnership within Judaism, encouraging Rivkah to provide support to her husband both in therapy and spiritually through prayer. This shift in perspective allowed her to redirect her focus from self-blame to recognizing herself as an integral part of the solution.

Since masturbation is forbidden within Orthodox Judaism, I needed to **find a creative solution** to deal with early ejaculation besides recommending masturbation before intercourse. With the permission of the couple, I contacted their rabbi to discuss my assessment of the couple and I explained to him the common known treatments for early ejaculation (including the start-stop method and the squeeze technique), I also shared with him ways that I have worked with Orthodox couples in the past regarding this issue, including receiving permission from the rabbi to allow for ejaculation on the outside of the vagina. To my surprise, the rabbi was very open to using the start-stop method, with Rivka manually stimulating her partner, although he encouraged David to ejaculate as closely to the vulva as possible.

With their rabbi's approval, the treatment plan went as follows. The couple would engage in regular sexual activity with each other, without placing emphasis on intercourse. Once again, **incorporating faith tradition** into the treatment method, I told David to focus on his partner's pleasure, something that is outlined in the Talmud. It was explained to the couple that this was a wonderful chance to explore and understand each other's bodies as well as their own. The shifting of focus from intercourse relieved a lot of anxiety for both partners.

Both partners were introduced to the start-stop method as a technique for addressing premature ejaculation. It was explained that this method involves pausing sexual stimulation when David feels close to ejaculation and resuming once the sensation subsides. To facilitate the implementation of the start-stop method, it was suggested that they engage in this practice when both partners are undressed, which interestingly created a connection to their faith traditions' teachings on partnered sex. This approach allowed for greater convenience, as if David needed to ejaculate, it could be done in close proximity to the vulva. By incorporating this technique into their intimate interactions, they were encouraged to explore and gradually extend the duration of their sexual encounters while managing David's ejaculation timing.

The following week the couple had reported that they had tried the technique several times throughout the week. They were exceptionally excited that they were able to connect intimately, despite the fact that penetration had still not occurred. However, they were enjoying the experience so much that they were both consistently initiating sexual activity, including multiple times within the same day. The guilt David felt from ejaculating outside of the vagina was partially lessened by understanding the biological functioning of his body and since permission was given by his spiritual authority. He did make an effort each time to ejaculate close to the vulva as was recommended.

After two weeks of implementing this treatment strategy, the couple shared the positive news that they were able to finally consummate their marriage. However, it was noted that David continued to experience premature ejaculation shortly after intercourse. Nevertheless, the couple remained profoundly encouraged by the significant progress they had made within such a short period. The fact that they were able to work together through the treatment process showcased their strong commitment and growing passion for each other. This notable transformation was evident, highlighting the positive impact of their collaborative efforts and the strengthening of their emotional and sexual connection.

Following three months of therapy, David and Rivka successfully achieved their treatment goals and were discharged from therapy. They were able to overcome the challenges that had previously hindered their ability to consummate their marriage, resolve David's issue with early ejaculation, and eliminate Rivka's feelings of rejection. The progress they made together allowed them to move forward with a renewed sense of intimacy and fulfillment in their relationship. Shortly after completing therapy, the couple informed me of the joyful news that they were expecting their first child. This was a remarkable testament to the positive changes they experienced and the significant impact their journey had on their overall well-being and future together.

Case Study 2 – Thomas and Julia

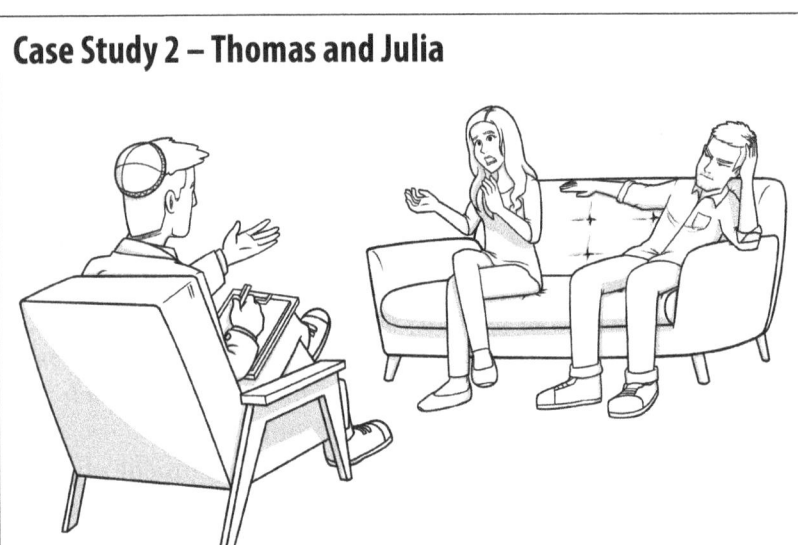

Thomas, 20, and Julia, 18, are both members of their local Southern Baptist Church. They recently got married in what Julia describes as her "dream wedding." The night of their wedding, Julia says that she was extremely nervous and decided it would be best to go slowly and begin by spending time in bed talking about sex. During that discussion, she discovered that Thomas was not a virgin and that he had had intercourse with two other partners. Julia felt betrayed and quickly got out of bed, put on her clothes, and locked herself in the bathroom, where she spent the night. She says she feels hurt and betrayed by Thomas and cannot believe that he did not keep himself pure for her. Thomas is speechless. He says that he loves Julia very much and never told her because he didn't want to hurt her and that the other girls meant nothing to him. He says he doesn't know what to do to make things better. Julia says that Thomas needs to repent and confess what he did in front of the church before she will consider moving forward. At the point of their initial intake session, the couple had not consummated their marriage.

Initial Interaction

Thomas took the initiative to schedule a therapy appointment, displaying evident confusion and a lack of understanding regarding Julia's response to their situation. While Thomas believed that God had forgiven him, he struggled to comprehend why Julia couldn't extend the same forgiveness. During the first session, I discovered that Julia had moved back in with her parents. She expressed her love for Thomas but labeled his actions as "cheating." When Thomas argued that it wasn't infidelity since they were not together at the time, Julia countered that his refusal to take responsibility indicated a lack of genuine repentance. The atmosphere between them was filled with hostility. Upon conducting my initial assessment, I recorded my impression that divorce might be the most viable option for the couple.

It was clear at the onset that neither Julia nor Thomas would have problems discussing the sexual issues that they were having. Even before the assessment properly began, Julia was ready to unload everything she thought about Thomas' past sexual behavior. However, even in these instances, the PLISSIT model is extremely important. While some patients may be okay with discussing certain aspects of sex and sexuality that they feel are relevant, they do not fully understand or grasp the full complexities and may not consider the connection to other areas outside of their presenting issue. Therefore, while asking for permission, I made it clear that we may be discussing topics outside of what they presented with in order to fully comprehend and assess their situation. In this case, both Julia and Thomas agreed.

Step 1 – Identify

In this unique case, the unconsummated marriage was not due to sexual dysfunction. Rather, one partner made the decision to abstain from physical intimacy upon discovering that their spouse had not remained celibate before marriage. Additionally, the high level of tension made communication difficult, limiting the possibility of the couple listening and understanding one another to reach a resolution.

Step 2 – Uncover

When exploring the couple's church teachings regarding sex and sexuality, it became apparent that their church subscribed to the principles of "Purity Culture." Purity Culture refers to a conservative religious framework that emphasizes abstinence before marriage and promotes strict sexual purity (Natarajan et al., 2022). It often includes teachings on maintaining virginity, modesty, and the belief that any sexual activity outside of marriage is morally wrong. Julia's perspective on sex was significantly influenced by growing up within this culture, which explains her intense reaction upon learning that Thomas was not a virgin. In contrast, Thomas's exposure to Purity Culture occurred later in his life when he began attending church at the age of 16. As a result, his beliefs and attitudes toward sex were not as deeply ingrained in the principles of purity culture as Julia's were.

Furthermore, it is important to consider that divorce may seem like the simplest solution due to the relatively short duration of their marriage. However, divorce is often strongly discouraged and even forbidden within some conservative Christian communities (Ademiluka, 2019). It is worth noting that in some conservative Christian churches, remarriage after divorce is not permitted, or at least viewed unfavorably (Li et al., 2018). Given that both partners were still young, pursuing divorce would not be a viable option for either of them. Considering the unfeasibility of divorce and the unique constraints they faced, I saw an opportunity to utilize this as motivation for the couple to actively engage in resolving their issues.

Step 3 – Recognize

When chairing a special interest group on sexuality and religion, I was able to gain insights into therapists' reactions to religion, particularly when it comes to strong negative sentiments. Often, these reactions stem from experiences related to purity culture. Many therapists have personal encounters within such environments that were profoundly negative. Considering the prevalence of purity culture within various church communities, it becomes challenging for individuals who grew up in such environments to separate purity culture from religion as a whole.

Given this context, it is understandable that a clinician might find themselves perplexed by Julia's response and instinctively lean towards siding with Thomas. However, it is imperative and ethically responsible to remain natural when working with couples. It is crucial for the clinician to acknowledge and validate Julia's feelings without hastily dismissing them. Recognizing and addressing her emotions will be essential in facilitating the couple's progress and moving forward in therapy.

Step 4 – Develop

At the onset of treatment, a crucial step was to provide the couple with a safe space to express their frustrations and feelings openly. It became evident that both partners carried significant internal conflicts, which greatly hindered their ability to listen and empathize with each other. The emotional turmoil within each of them created barriers to effective communication, making it challenging for them to find common ground and understanding.

During the initial sessions, I encouraged them to share their perspectives without interruption or judgment, allowing their emotions to be fully acknowledged and validated. This process proved to be cathartic for the couple individually, as they were able to release pent-up emotions and gain clarity about their own feelings and thought processes. This also provided me the opportunity to employ a technique that would allow the couple to begin working together, fighting for their marriage instead of against each other. I made a deliberate comment that sought to challenge their negative perceptions of each other.

I shared with the couple that in my assessment notes, I had written that divorce seemed like a plausible solution for them, given their low opinions of each other and apparent unwillingness to work through their issues. I mentioned, "You know, since both of you seem to hold such low opinions of each other and appear unwilling to work through this, perhaps that is the right assessment. It would be easier, and I can't think of a single reason why the two of you should stay together." This statement aimed to provoke a reaction and initiate a shift in their dynamic, challenging them to confront the reality of their situation.

This was also an opportunity to **incorporate their faith tradition** as part of a **creative solution** for their situation. As divorce conflicted with their religious beliefs, both Julia and Thomas swiftly rejected the idea. It was something that neither were willing to consider. Their rejection of the idea became a turning point in the therapeutic process, prompting them to reflect on the reasons why they loved each other and desired to remain married. This led to a deeper exploration of their core values and beliefs.

As both partners expressed their feelings about the other, I said to Julia, "If you love Thomas so much, what's the problem? Why can't you just forgive him and move on?" This question allowed us to delve gradually into the underlying beliefs and values that shaped her reactions.

I told her, "Now that you've shared with me what your faith teaches *against* but tell me what your faith teaches *about* compassion and forgiveness." This provided another opportunity for the couple to incorporate their faith tradition into the therapeutic process. Julia acknowledged that forgiveness and compassion were essential components to her faith, yet stated that she was unsure how to move past knowing that he had engaged in sexual activity and forgive him, especially since her church has such strong teachings against what he had done.

We acknowledged the role of these ingrained beliefs, opening the door for **psychosexual education** that focused on sexual health and wellness, while also respecting their religious beliefs. Both partners were informed about sexual development throughout the lifespan and healthy sexual behavior. This led me to ask Julia if she would feel more comfortable if Thomas was tested for STIs and HIV, to which she nodded in agreement. She stated that this would provide her with some comfort, knowing that their sexual engagement would be safe.

During this time in therapy, I also helped the couples to develop more effective communication skills. This process of emotional expression and introspection laid the foundation for the next phase of therapy, which focused on facilitating constructive dialogue and promoting mutual understanding. We worked on developing effective communication skills, active listening techniques, and empathy-building exercises. These tools empowered the couple to communicate their needs, fears, and desires more openly and honestly, fostering deeper connections and empathy for each other's experiences.

As therapy progressed, both Julia and Thomas gained a better understanding of how their past experiences and religious teachings had influenced their present conflicts. Julia gradually shifted her perspective, recognizing that her judgments were heavily influenced by the expectations imposed by Purity Culture. Thomas, on the other hand, learned to empathize with Julia's emotions and acknowledge the significance of her religious background in shaping her beliefs.

Around the fifth month of therapy, as trust and healthy communication skills developed, the couple felt ready to engage in sexual interaction, marking an important milestone in their journey. With ongoing support and guidance, they eventually consummated their marriage. After seven months of treatment, the couple reached their treatment goals and were discharged from therapy, having consummated their marriage, resolved relational conflicts, and gained greater respect and appreciation for one another.

Case Study 3 – Omar and Aisha

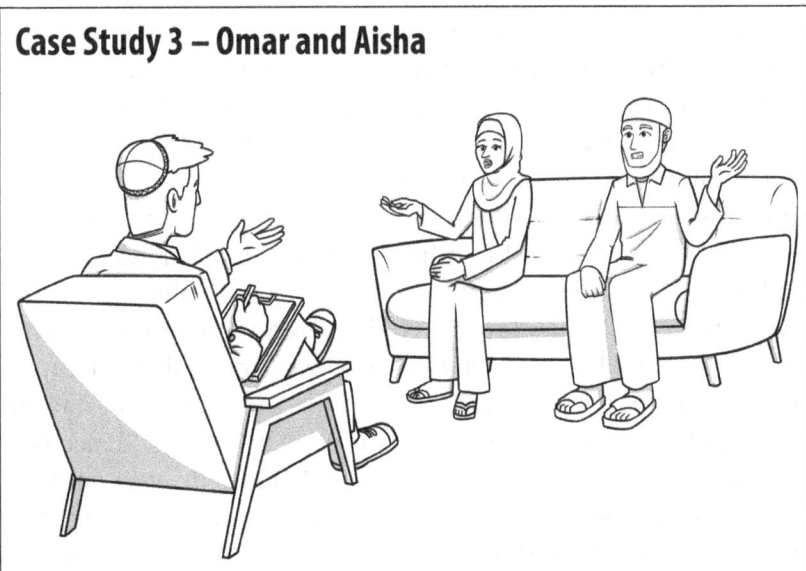

Omar, 22, and Aisha, 20, were brought up in a very conservative and religious Islamic environment. Although their families arranged their marriage, they both agreed to it. However, on their wedding night, Aisha felt extremely anxious and "froze up." She experienced unbearable pain when Omar tried to penetrate her, and he was unable to do so. Concerned, Aisha went to see her OBGYN, who could not find any medical explanation for her pain. Despite this, Aisha decided to try again, but the experience was the same – she experienced severe pain, and Omar was unable to penetrate. Omar was terrified that he was causing his wife harm and felt guilty for his inability to have intercourse with her. The couple has since decided to avoid attempting intercourse altogether. However, due to their religious beliefs concerning consummating the marriage and the importance of family, they have come to sex therapy with hopes of resolving the issue and helping them to have a "normal" sex life.

Initial Interaction

Both Omar and Aisha exhibited signs of nervousness and apprehension during their initial assessment, which can be attributed to their young age and lack of understanding and experience in matters of human sexual function. Their timid demeanor and hesitancy to discuss their sexual issues indicated their discomfort in addressing this sensitive topic. To help alleviate their anxiety and create a more relaxed atmosphere, I often utilized humor as a means to foster a safe space for open dialogue. This also became the moment to introduce the PLISSIT model.

When asking the couple for permission to discuss sexual issues, the couple displayed avoidance and appeared to agree reluctantly, possibly out of a desire to please me as their therapist rather than giving genuine consent. Sensing their hesitation, I decided to address their concerns directly by saying, "It seemed both of you were a bit hesitant to agree. How do you actually feel about talking about these topics?" They both expressed nervousness and revealed that they had never discussed sexual issues with anyone before. I reassured them that their comfort was paramount, and if they ever felt uncomfortable, they could simply let me know. I emphasized that I did not want them to engage in or discuss anything beyond their comfort zone. Understanding their apprehension, I planned to revisit these topics when they appeared more at ease discussing sex. However, with this understanding and assurance, both patients' apprehension diminished over time, and after one month of therapy, they became much more comfortable discussing sex with both me and their partner.

Early on, it became apparent that both Omar and Aisha carried a sense of responsibility for their unconsummated marriage. They believed that by avoiding sexual intimacy, they could wait for a natural progression where the issue would resolve itself without causing further complications. However, upon the recommendation of Aisha's aunt, they were willing to embark on the journey of sex therapy, displaying a willingness to address and resolve their sexual challenges.

Step 1 – Identify

The couple sought therapy due to their unconsummated marriage. After conducting an assessment, it became clear that Aisha was experiencing pain during penetration, which was indicative of a condition called vaginismus. This condition is traditionally described as involuntary muscle contractions in the pelvic floor, caused by actual or anticipated pain during sexual intercourse (Laskowska & Gronowski, 2022). Consequently, Omar felt a sense of responsibility for causing his wife pain, and as a result, both partners started avoiding intimacy altogether to prevent further discomfort and emotional distress.

Step 2 – Uncover

The importance of family within Islam adds a significant weight to the challenges faced by the couple due to their inability to consummate their marriage. In this particular case, vaginismus is likely connected to the difficulties experienced by some religious women when transitioning from a period of actively refraining from sexual behavior to engaging in it (Aktan Mutlu & Koc, 2021). These findings align with a study conducted in 2008, which revealed that 81% of unconsummated cases in a Muslim country were attributed to vaginismus (Ozdemir et al., 2008). The anxiety associated with fulfilling this new role often exacerbates the severity of the condition, further impacting the couple's well-being and marital satisfaction.

Furthermore, within Islamic teachings, there are instructions for men to treat their wives with kindness and care (Al-Tirmidhi, 3895; Ibn Majah, 1977). It is reasonable to consider that Omar's sense of blame is somewhat influenced by his religious beliefs, as he may feel a deep responsibility to uphold these teachings. Research conducted on Muslim couples in Iran has shown that many men experience significant distress and fear when they believe they are causing their wives pain, to the extent that their responses resemble symptoms of post-traumatic stress disorder (Bokaie et al., 2017). This highlights the severity of the condition for both partners and emphasizes the importance of addressing the issue in a holistic manner that respects their religious beliefs and values.

Step 3 – Recognize

In this specific case, there are no specific religious teachings that can be identified as directly causing the couple's sexual issues. However, the clinician may hold personal beliefs that consider the patient's religious beliefs as outdated or unnecessary. It is important to acknowledge that while specific religious teachings may not be the cause, the couple's overall religious devotion does contribute to their sexual issue. Despite any reservations, it is important for the clinician to recognize that the couple's religious tradition plays a significant role in fostering the husband's unwavering support and active involvement in helping his wife receive the best possible care. Moreover, their religious tradition emphasizes the importance of their relationship. Therefore, rather than focusing on singling out problematic teachings, clinicians should emphasize the positive elements of their patient's faith and incorporate those elements into the therapeutic process.

Step 4 – Develop

Research on Muslim couples facing unconsummated marriages as a result of vaginismus suggests a comprehensive approach to treatment. This multidimensional approach includes various methods such as narrative exposure therapy, providing education on the anatomy of the female and male reproductive systems, correcting misconceptions, educating on the importance of foreplay, guiding the exploration of the body through non-sexual and sexual massage, and gradually progressing to penetration starting with the woman's finger and then the man's after achieving relaxation (Bokaie et al., 2017).

Psychosexual education played a crucial role in this treatment approach. Providing comprehensive knowledge about the anatomy of the female and male reproductive systems was essential for dispelling misconceptions and fostering a better understanding of sexual health and functioning (Hosseini et al., 2017). Correcting any misinformation or cultural beliefs that may perpetuate anxiety or fear surrounding sexual intercourse was vital in helping couples develop a more positive and informed mindset (Aliabadian et al., 2020).

Foreplay education was included as part of the psychosexual education. The couple was guided in understanding the significance of foreplay in arousal and relaxation, as it can play a pivotal role in overcoming vaginismus. By focusing on sensual and non-penetrative activities, such as body exploration and non-sexual and sexual massage, the couple was able to gradually cultivate a sense of trust, relaxation, and pleasure in the sexual context.

It was also essential to **incorporate their religious tradition** within the therapeutic process. This was done by throughout the therapeutic process as I often checked with the couple concerning how they thought their religious beliefs informed their commitment to each other and efforts in overcoming the sexual dysfunction. It was also prevalent in narrative exposure therapy, where I focused on religiously informed values. Thus, it became part of the **creative solutions** that we initiated within the therapeutic alliance.

To address the specific issue of penetration, a gradual and step-by-step approach was used. Initially, Aisha was encouraged to explore her own body and become comfortable with self-penetration using their her fingers. This self-exploration allows women to gain control over their bodies and experience relaxation.

However, Aisha was not entirely comfortable with this idea at first, therefore, I suggested the use of dilators, which to her, felt like a more medical solution that she was willing to engage with. Eventually, I helped the couple progress to using Omar's fingers, gradually working towards successful penetration.

After four months in therapy, the couple finally consummated their marriage. The simple relief of finally consummating the marriage reduced the distress and anxiety felt by both partners, which in turn helped reduce any remaining discomfort Aisha felt during penetration. As suggested by the research, the couple was asked to follow up a month later, where the couple showed further improvement in their sexual functioning and reported an increase in marital satisfaction (Bokaie et al., 2017).

Conclusion

Unconsummated marriages continue to be a significant issue, particularly within religious and culturally conservative communities. Despite evolving definitions of sex and changing societal norms, the prevalence of unconsummated marriages remains evident. Religious leaders often recommend seeking the help of sex therapists in resolving this issue, emphasizing the importance of addressing it within the context of faith and spirituality (Friedman, 2019).

Factors contributing to unconsummated marriages are diverse, ranging from insufficient sexual knowledge to anxiety, cultural expectations, and specific sexual dysfunctions (Hosseini et al., 2017; Laskowska & Gronowski, 2022). Vaginismus, dyspareunia, premature ejaculation, and erectile dysfunction are common factors that hinder the establishment of a fulfilling sexual relationship (Ozdemir et al., 2008). The consequences of unconsummated marriages can be severe, including feelings of guilt, shame, inadequacy, strained relationships, and increased risk of divorce.

Cultural and religious influences play a significant role in shaping individuals' experiences of unconsummated marriages

(Ribner & Rosenbaum, 2005; Aktan Mutlu & Koc, 2021). The pressure to conform to societal expectations, preserve virginity, and adhere to rigid sexual norms can create immense anxiety and make the transition into sexual intimacy challenging. Cultural and religious expectations often emphasize purity and place a burden on individuals to navigate complex sexual dynamics within these constraints.

Addressing unconsummated marriages requires a comprehensive approach that recognizes the multifaceted nature of the issue (Bokaie et al., 2017; Xi et al., 2023). Providing accurate sexual education, fostering open communication, addressing psychological factors, and challenging restrictive cultural and religious beliefs are essential components of effective treatment. By considering the physical, psychological, religious, and cultural dimensions, clinicians can help individuals and couples navigate the challenges, alleviate guilt and shame, and work towards establishing a satisfying and intimate relationship all while fostering a fulfilling and intimate connection within the context of their religious beliefs and values.

References

Ademiluka, S. O. (2019). "For I hate divorce," says the Lord: Interpreting Malachi 2:16 in relation to prohibition of divorce in some churches in Nigeria. *Old Testament Essays*, *32*(3), 846–868. DOI: 10.17159/2312–3621/2019/v32n3a5

Aktan Mutlu, E., & Koc, M. (2021). The role of religiosity in the etiology of vaginismus in the light of socio-cultural features: The case of Turkey. *Dicle Tıp Dergisi*, *48*(3), 404–415. DOI: 10.5798/dicletip.987807

Aliabadian, A., Hassanzadeh, R., & Mirzaian, B. (2020). Effectiveness of couples' sexual training on marital quality, sexual attitude, and knowledge of women in unconsummated marriage. *Journal of Nursing and Midwifery Sciences*, *7*(3), 139–145. DOI: 10.4103/JNMS. JNMS_57_19

Alla, S. R. (2017). 351 clinical profile of unconsummated marriages. *Journal of Sexual Medicine*, *14*(1), S103. DOI: 10.1016/j.jsxm.2016.11.238

Bokaie, M., Khalesi, Z. B., & Yasini-Ardekani, S. M. (2017). Diagnosis and treatment of unconsummated marriage in an Iranian couple. *African Health Sciences, 17*(3), 623–636. DOI: 10.4314/ahs.v17i3.5

Friedman, S. (2019). Assessing and treating sexual dysfunctions in Orthodox Jewish couples: A summary of 41 consecutive cases. *Mental Health, Religion & Culture, 22*(9), 930–942. DOI: 10.1080/13674676.2019.1688269

Hosseini, S., Noroozi, M., & Montazery, G. (2017). Investigating the relation between women's body image and unconsummated marriage. *Iranian Journal of Nursing and Midwifery Research, 22*(5), 363–366. DOI: 10.4103/ijnmr.IJNMR_176_16

Kojo, K., Oda, H., Suetomi, T., Negoro, H., & Nishiyama, H. (2022). A review of intravaginal ejaculatory dysfunction and unconsummated marriage cases in the outpatient clinic for male infertility at the University of Tsukuba hospital. *Journal of Sexual Medicine, 19*(5), S206. DOI: 10.1016/j.jsxm.2022.03.468

Laskowska, A., & Gronowski, P. (2022). Vaginismus: An overview. *Journal of Sexual Medicine, 19*(5), S228–S229. DOI: 10.1016/j.jsxm.2022.03.520

Li, S., Kubzansky, L. D., & VanderWeele, T. J. (2018). Religious service attendance, divorce, and remarriage among U.S. nurses in mid and late life. *PloS One, 13*(12), e0207778–e0207778. DOI: 10.1371/journal.pone.0207778

Mohamed Mohamed, E., Abdel-Aleem, H., & Hamdy, A. (2021). Assessment of sexual dysfunctions among newly married couples in Egypt: A case-control study. *Al-Azhar Assist Medical Journal: AAMJ, 19*(4), 560–563. DOI: 10.4103/azmj.azmj_10_21

Natarajan, M., Wilkins-Yel, K. G., Sista, A., Anantharaman, A., & Seils, N. (2022). Decolonizing purity culture: Gendered racism and white idealization in evangelical Christianity. *Psychology of Women Quarterly, 46*(3), 316–336. DIO: 10.1177/03616843221091116

Ozdemir, O., Simsek, F., Ozkardes, S., Incesu, C., & Karakoc, B. (2008). The unconsummated marriage: Its frequency and clinical characteristics in a sexual dysfunction clinic. *Journal of Sex & Marital Therapy, 34*(3), 268–279. DOI: 10.1080/00926230701866380

Ribner, D. S., & Rosenbaum, T. Y. (2005). Evaluation and treatment of unconsummated marriages among orthodox Jewish couples. *Journal of Sex & Marital Therapy, 31*(4), 341–353. DOI: 10.1080/00926230590950244

Xi, Y., Xia, T., Colonnello, E., Wang, C., Lai, Y., & Zhang, Y. (2023). Unconsummated marriage among Chinese couples: A retrospective study. *Sexual Medicine*, *11*(1), qfac003. DOI: 10.1093/sexmed/qfac003

Zargooshi, J. (2008). Male sexual dysfunction in unconsummated marriage: Long-term outcome in 417 patients. *Journal of Sexual Medicine*, *5*(12), 2895–2903. DOI: 10.1111/j.1743–6109.2008.01004.x

10

Mixed and Intrareligious Marriages

Introduction

Our sexual values inform who we are, the way that we think about sex, and the way in which we approach our sexual partners. Conflict can arise when one partner's sexual values are different from those of their partner. As with all values, our sexual values have been informed by numerous spheres of influence, including our family of origin and, in many cases, religion. Previous chapters have addressed the way Judaism, Christianity, and Islam view sex and the boundaries that each faith group has established around sexual activity. Differences in thoughts can be seen within each faith tradition, as well as in comparison of one faith tradition to the other. These differences can lead to sexual problems within a marriage due to the partners holding differing values and boundaries around sex.

Religious difference is often highlighted as the primary conflictual dimension of a relationship in academic literature (Cerchiaro, 2020). There are two ways in which religious differences can be present in the therapy room:[1]

1. **Interreligious**, or **mixed-faith marriages** are unions in which each partner belongs to a different religious tradition. Couples finding themselves in the early stages of

DOI: 10.4324/9781003242017-14

marriage not only have difficulty navigating cohabit-ation as newlyweds but also the complex terrain of sexu-ality when their partner holds different beliefs about sex and the role of sex in the relationship. Examples of an interreligious marriage include a Muslim married to a Buddhist, or a Christian married to a Jew. The conflict of an interreligious marriage also includes navigating different faith traditions and communities, as well as discussions around procreation and the heritage that will be passed down to their offspring.

2. **Intrareligious marriages** are those in which each partner is a part of the same religious tradition but belongs to a different sect or denomination. I also use this term to describe couples who may be in the same sect or denom-ination but where one partner becomes less observant than the other. Examples of intrareligious marriage include a Southern Baptist Christian married to a Roman Catholic, or an Orthodox Jew married to a Reform Jew. Couples in intrareligious marriages often experience a phenomenon where one partner assumes that their denomination or sect is superior or the proper way to live out their faith tradition.

Both Orthodox Judaism and conservative Christianity discourage interreligious marriages. Typically, if the partner is from outside of their faith tradition, they would require them to convert. For example, if an Orthodox Jewish woman met a man who was not Jewish, it would most likely be required that he convert in order for the marriage to take place. Islam, on the other hand, allows interreligious marriages under certain conditions. It is generally accepted that a Muslim man can marry a woman who is either Jewish or Christian; although the same allowance is not typically given to Muslim women (Ramadan, 2017, 182).

Therapist Bias Check

1. Am I making assumptions about the couple's beliefs or behaviors based on my own personal beliefs or experiences with their religion or faith background?

2. Am I being respectful and non-judgmental towards both partners' beliefs and practices, or am I favoring one partner's beliefs over the other?

Case Study 1 – Levi and Savannah

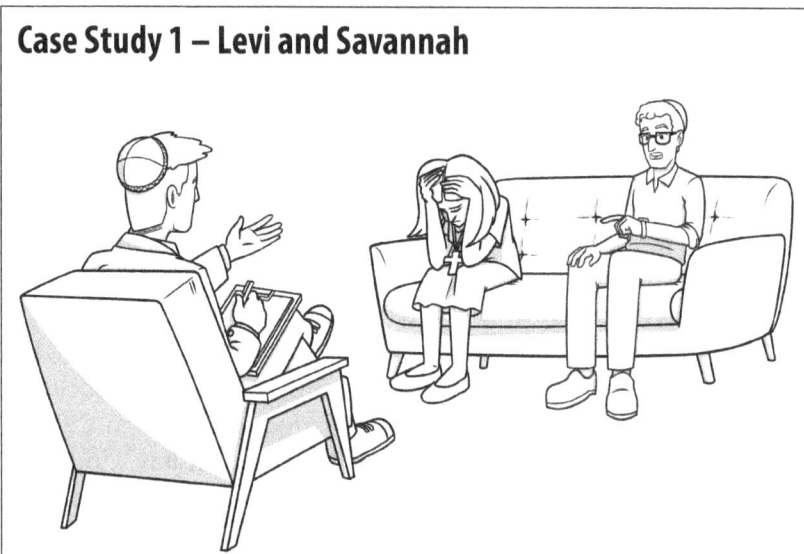

Savannah, a 23-year-old graduate student from a Catholic background, and Levi, her 24-year-old husband, have been married for six months. Levi grew up as an Orthodox Jew, but he describes his family as less religious. The couple met in high school, during a period when Levi was rebelling against his family and faith. They dated for a few years, and while they participated in each other's faith traditions, Levi eventually proposed to Savannah on the condition that he would convert to Catholicism.

After their wedding, however, Levi began to feel doubts about his decision to convert. Despite his love for Savannah, he told her that he couldn't live his life as a Catholic. This confession devastated Savannah, who reminded him that Catholics didn't believe in divorce. Levi suggested two options: they could stay married but not have children, or Savannah could convert to Judaism so they could have children and stay married. Feeling overwhelmed, Savannah decided to move out and has been considering divorce. The couple's religious differences have put a strain on their relationship, and they are struggling to find a way forward that honors both of their faiths while also preserving their love and commitment to each other.

Initial Interaction

In contrast to other couples who enter therapy and may initially mask relationship issues, Savannah's evident negative emotions toward her partner were palpable upon their arrival. Her tone and communication reflected these sentiments from the outset. During the session, as I introduced the framework of sex therapy using the PLISSIT model, I sought explicit permission from both individuals to engage in discussions related to sexuality, to which they both consented. Given the existing tension between them, I encouraged not only self-permission but also mutual permission to discuss intimate matters. Additionally, I emphasized the importance of maintaining respect for each other's perspectives and feelings surrounding sexuality.

Savannah showed no willingness to discuss the subject of their marriage with an open mind or compromise in order to salvage their marriage. In her mind, the only options were for Levi to remain a Catholic and for them to have children, or to end their marriage. She failed to acknowledge Levi's spiritual struggle and dismissed his theological opinions by citing New Testament scripture, without attempting to understand or empathize with his perspective. Levi appeared somewhat at a crossroads where his only choices were to be authentic to himself and embrace his Judaism or reject his heritage to be with the woman he loved since high school.

Step 1 – Identify

In this particular case study, Levi's decision to abandon Catholicism and return to Judaism was the primary issue. He attempted to propose a compromise to Savannah, suggesting three options: (1) they could remain married without having children, (2) she could convert to Judaism, or (3) they could opt for a divorce. Both partners were deeply hurt and felt betrayed by one another due to the religious discussions they had after getting married. For Savannah, this was a topic they had discussed prior to their marriage, and she couldn't understand why Levi would backpedal on his premarital commitments. Additionally, she struggled to accept his abandonment of Catholicism. Conversely, Levi believed that Savannah was trying to impose her religious beliefs on him, and he was hurt by her unwillingness to view things from his spiritual perspective.

Step 2 – Uncover

Savannah and Levi's religious teachings and beliefs create a complex dynamic in their marriage, making their situation particularly challenging. Savannah's Christian background, rooted in Catholicism, emphasizes the importance of faith in Jesus Christ and the sanctity of marriage as a lifelong commitment. The Catholic doctrine strongly discourages divorce, aligning with the broader Christian principle that marriage is a sacred union ordained by God (Matthew 19:6, English Standard Version). This perspective underscores Savannah's deep commitment to her Christian faith and her desire for a marriage that adheres to Christian values.

On the other hand, Levi's Orthodox Jewish principles bring a distinct set of challenges to the relationship. Within Orthodox Judaism, Jewish identity encompasses not only religious beliefs but also cultural and ethnic elements. The process of conversion to Judaism is rigorous, involving comprehensive study, ritual immersion, and adherence to Jewish law and customs. Levi's initial decision to convert to Catholicism and his subsequent doubts about this conversion reflect a complex journey of religious identity. His Orthodox Jewish background places a strong emphasis on preserving Jewish heritage, and Jewish identity is traditionally passed down through the mother's line.

The interplay of these contrasting religious teachings creates a profound dilemma for the couple. Savannah's commitment to her Christian faith and her expectation of a Catholic marriage may seem incompatible with Levi's desire to reconnect with his Jewish heritage. The prospect of having children further complicates matters, as it raises questions about how to instill religious values in their future family while honoring their individual faith traditions. These religious teachings form the backdrop against which Savannah and Levi must navigate their relationship, seeking a path that respects their respective faiths while preserving their love and commitment to each other.

Step 3 – Recognize

In the case of Levi and Savannah, a complex web of potential biases can emerge, presenting intricate challenges to the therapeutic process and the therapist's objectivity. Among therapists, there may be a tendency to align with Levi's perspective, perceiving Savannah as overbearing or unreasonable in her attitudes toward Levi and his autonomy. This partiality may become even more pronounced when the therapist shares a Jewish background, raising personal objections to Savannah's persistence that Levi leave Judaism for Christianity. Furthermore, for an Orthodox clinician, Levi's initial contemplation of conversion might trigger surprise or confusion, subtly influencing their perception of him. Conversely, a Christian therapist, particularly one with a fundamentalist or evangelical background, may grapple with an internal impulse to endorse the concept of conversion, driven by their faith-based convictions. They may also harbor negative sentiments toward Levi's decision to leave Christianity and return to Judaism, potentially biasing their judgment in favor of advocating for her separation from Levi. In these intricate scenarios, clinicians must navigate the intricate balance of maintaining impartiality while diligently guarding against the encroachment of their personal opinions and beliefs, all in the pursuit of fostering a truly unbiased therapeutic process.

Step 4 – Develop

To be frank, by the end of the initial session, my professional opinion was that it may be in the best interest of both Savannah and Levi to end their marriage. Despite their long-standing relationship throughout high school, the couple had only been married for six months, and I thought it best they end the relationship before investing any more time or energy. Both were pursuing master's degrees, albeit in different subjects, and it seemed reasonable that they could focus on their chosen field instead of struggling with convincing the other to change their mind.

Nevertheless, the couple seemed extremely desperate, partially because they were far from home and without a support system, so I agreed to work with them

In this particular case, **psychosexual education** Was not needed, nor would it have an effective role in the therapeutic process. Both of the partners were well aware of body functioning and sexual functioning, as indicated on the intake form. They also stated that neither of them had questions about their bodies or about sexuality. Therefore, in this particular instance, there is no need to think that psychosexual education would have been beneficial. By both partner's accounts, their sex life had always been good and was one of the reasons that they had decided to get married.

As with all religious couples, I try to find creative ways to **incorporate their faith tradition** into the clinical setting. The goal in this instance is to find out where each partner is concerning their spiritual beliefs and how they relate and impact their marriage. In this instance, there was a discrepancy, Levi, as a Jew, did not find divorce to be wrong or sinful, whereas Savannah's Catholic faith taught her that divorce was wrong regardless of the circumstances. Yet, in this particular instance, it seemed that Levi was more willing to find ways to compromise in order to make their relationship work, whereas Savannah was willing to consider divorce.

Savannah appeared to be experiencing cognitive dissonance, so I probed her about her thoughts on divorce despite her church's teachings against it in order to help her find some congruency. She explained that Levi's false conversion was a betrayal of faith and family, and felt that marrying someone of the same faith who was a strong Christian leader was essential. She insisted on raising her children in a religious household and found all of Levi's suggestions for compromise to be inadequate. Savannah believed that marrying an unbeliever was her biggest sin, for which she consistently sought God's forgiveness. She attributed her decision to marry Levi to losing her virginity to him before they were married and acknowledged that it was not a rational choice.

Additionally, Savannah had the belief that if Levi actually loved her he would make such a drastic alteration in his life. She refused to accept the fact that his faith tradition and family history could have any relevance to him. In her mind, she was offering him something much better and the decision should be simple, in fact she stated that Levi, "shouldn't have to think about it." While she considered Levi's denial of Catholicism a statement of his love and commitment to her, she did not acknowledge how her lack of willingness to compromise demonstrated to Levi her lack of affection for him. This left Levi very surprised and hurt as he realized that his partner did not value him the same way that he valued her.

Both Savannah and Levi had moved to the UK three months after they were married in order to attend university. While they were both in separate degree programs and in separate departments, they were attending the same university, meaning that they would occasionally see each other. They had no support system, since all of their family and friends were back in the United States. Even more complicated, is that both partners had to discover ways of handling housing since Savannah decided to move out on her own when she separated from Levi. This created a financial strain on both of them.

While it seemed that there was little that could be done to salvage the marriage since Savannah was pretty adamant on ending the relationship if Levi did not remain Catholic, I thought it best for all involved if we **found creative solutions** to make the separation as amiable as possible. To begin this process, I asked the couple what they thought would be the biggest difficulties that they would face should they separate. The list between the two were similar. Savannah was worried about finances and what her family and friends would think for her to not only divorce but to be married for such a short period of time. Levi was concerned with finding stable housing and how to break the news to his parents. Both were concerned with being alone in a foreign country.

Savannah and Levi had both expressed concerns and fear about being alone in a foreign country if they were to divorce. Despite this, both partners agreed that they wanted to stay in the UK to pursue their education and enjoy the opportunity to study abroad. In response to their concerns, I provided them with several solutions to help them establish a support system and gain more friends. For Savannah, who had a passion for singing, I suggested finding local choirs to join either at the university or through Christian organizations. I also recommended that she become more involved in a local church to build connections with other members of the community. For Levi, I advised finding a local synagogue where he could connect with the Jewish community, and getting involved in Jewish groups on campus like Hillel. I also recommended that both would benefit from checking with the university's international office to find out about student activities and events where they could connect with others, including other Americans who may be studying there.

While therapy is not the ideal setting to tackle financial and housing concerns, I recognized the importance of regularly checking in with Savannah and Levi regarding their financial stability and housing search. To instill a sense of accountability, I made it a point to ask for updates during each therapy session. Additionally, at the end of each session, when setting goals for the week, I would incorporate this discussion to help them stay focused on their financial and housing objectives for the week. This was an attempt to reduce stress and anxiety on behalf of both partners which could interfere with the work we were doing in therapy.

To help the couple navigate their family dynamics, I found it necessary to address how they would communicate the state of their relationship to their families. Both Savannah and Levi's parents were worried about the status of their relationship, but felt unable to help since they were far away. At first, we practiced healthy and respectful ways for them to communicate to their parents that they were not comfortable discussing their relationship situation, but informed them that they were seeking couple's therapy to resolve certain issues. As time went on, it became clear that it would be beneficial to help them find ways to tell their parents that they would be separating and ending their relationship. Although this was a difficult task, I assigned them a joint homework assignment to write a letter to their parents explaining their decision. This would give them a script to use during a phone or in-person conversation with their parents. For the assignment, I encouraged the couple to ask each other for help and work together should the task prove difficult.

The following week, Savannah and Levi walked into my office and immediately, I noticed a change in their demeanor. They seemed more relaxed and open with one another. As we began our session, they informed me that they had completed the homework assignment that I had given them, which was to write a letter to their parents informing them of their decision to end their relationship. They told me that while it was difficult to write the letters, they were grateful that they could work on the assignment together. They found it very helpful to have the support of the other.

During the session, I noticed that the two were interacting with each other in a more positive and collaborative manner than they had in previous sessions. This was the first time in the therapeutic process that the two worked as partners and there was a noticeable decrease in hostility toward one another. In fact, it was noticeable that underneath the hurt and resentment the two were very good friends, and it was my hope that that. while the relationship most likely would end, the friendship would be salvageable.

We spent the session with each reading the letter that they had written, while the other acting as though they were the parent listening. This was a very moving moment for each and both Savannah and Levi cried during this role play. It was clear that this exercise was a bonding moment for the two. We also discussed ways to further develop their friendship outside of the romantic relationship. The progress that Savannah and Levi made in this session gave me hope that they could move forward in a positive direction and that they would be able to navigate their separation in a healthy way.

After several months of therapy, it became clear that Savannah and Levi were not willing to meet each other's terms. Although Levi expressed his love for Savannah and regret that they were unable to find a compromise that would make both of them happy, Savannah remained bitter and could not understand why Levi did not want to become Catholic. She felt like she wasn't enough for him to want to embrace her faith. Despite the Church's teaching on divorce, Savannah ultimately made the difficult decision to leave her husband and pursue a divorce.

However, it was not all bleak for the couple. Through therapy, they had discovered ways to improve their communication and agreed to offer support to one another if ever needed. While their marriage had come to an end, they both recognized the importance of maintaining a healthy relationship for the sake of their own emotional well-being and any potential future interactions. It was my hope that they would be able to move forward and find happiness in their individual journeys.

Case Study 2 – Ishaaq and Naomi

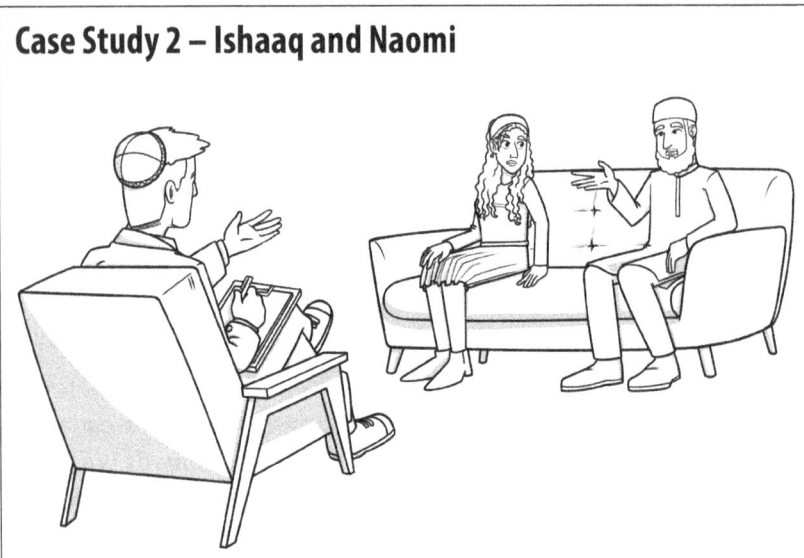

Ishaaq, a 31-year-old Muslim man, and Naomi, a 27-year-old Jewish woman, got married recently, both claiming that religion didn't play a significant role in their upbringing, although it remains an essential part of their identity. They expressed their love for each other and how happy they were being married. After a year and a half of marriage, Naomi found out that she was pregnant, and both she and Ishaaq were thrilled. They informed their parents, who were equally happy, but their ideas for the child's future were different.

Ishaaq's family was overjoyed to be expecting a Muslim grandchild and wanted the child to be raised traditionally with Naomi staying home to care for the child. Naomi's family, on the other hand, was hoping for a boy and wanted to arrange a *brit milah* (ceremonial circumcision of a male infant, performed when the baby is eight days old), and had already begun searching for Jewish daycares for when Naomi returned to work. The pressure and confusion from both families have caused significant conflicts in their relationship. Ishaaq believes his parents' opinion is correct, while Naomi insists that her parents are correct and that they will follow their lead. The couple admits to fighting regularly for the first time in their relationship, and they have decided not to have any more children if they do stay together and will no longer be intimate.

Initial Interaction

Upon meeting Ishaaq and Naomi, it was evident that both were well-educated and came from affluent families, as indicated by their language, clothing, and demeanor. However, despite their privileged backgrounds, it was clear that the couple was struggling with relationship issues caused by their differing religious beliefs. They appeared unprepared for the challenges of navigating their first child's upbringing while dealing with a clash of religious opinions. As they spoke, there was a sense of tension and unease in their interactions, with both partners nitpicking each other's words and resorting to making subtle jabs and snide remarks. As I introduced the PLISSIT model, I emphasized the aspect of each partner not only granting permission for the other to discuss sex, but being respectful of what the other shares.

In addition to the challenges posed by their differing religious beliefs, the couple was also struggling to navigate the impact that their families' views were having on their relationship. With each partner feeling a strong sense of loyalty and obligation to their respective families, tensions began to rise as they felt increasingly caught in the middle of a familial tug-of-war. As discussions became more heated, both Ishaaq and Naomi felt compelled to defend their parents' beliefs, leading to a further breakdown in communication between the couple. At the same time, they felt personally attacked by the other's family, leading to feelings of resentment and hurt. This added layer of complexity only served to exacerbate the already difficult situation they were facing.

Step 1 – Identify

Simply put, the couple had neglected to have a conversation about the role of religion and religious practices in their family, particularly when it came to raising children. As a Muslim, Isaaq had a different fundamental understanding of what would happen when he and his partner had a child and the way that child would be raised, than Naomi who was influenced by her Jewish tradition. Unfortunately, neither partner was willing to make concessions, citing their religious conviction.

Step 2 – Uncover

Although both Ishaaq and Naomi belonged to an Abrahamic faith, they were confronted with the realization that their religious traditions held contrasting views regarding family and religious heritage. According to Islamic law, the religion is passed down through the father, which means that a Muslim man can marry a woman from the Jewish or Christian faith since the child would still be considered Muslim (Ramadan, 2017, 182). In contrast, Judaism transmits its religion through the mother, meaning that a person is only considered Jewish if their mother is Jewish, or they have gone through an acceptable conversion (Baskin, 1998, 3–20; Lehman et al., 2017).

These differing worldviews on the transmission of religion became a source of contention for the couple, as they were both unprepared to compromise on their beliefs. Additionally, neither partner had discussed the place of religion and religious practices in their family, particularly with regard to their future children. They both assumed that their child would inherit their religious identity, without recognizing that the other partner's faith tradition taught something entirely different. This lack of communication and understanding only served to exacerbate the issue and widen the gap between the couple.

Step 3 – Recognize
Working with Ishaaq and Naomi, therapists should be vigilant about various potential biases that may emerge, influencing the therapeutic dynamics. A non-religious therapist, for instance, might perceive the worldviews of both partners as antiquated or outdated, potentially leading to offense regarding their perspectives on gender roles within the marital relationship. A Muslim clinician could find it easier to empathize with Ishaaq than Naomi, while a Jewish therapist may naturally align more closely with Naomi and express objections to Ishaaq's standpoint. In these intricate situations, the risk of harboring hostility toward one or both patients is palpable, potentially triggering a defensive response from the therapist. This underscores the importance of therapists remaining vigilant in addressing these biases to maintain an objective therapeutic environment.

Step 4 – Develop
In this particular case, the path toward congruency was not with the individual's faith and their sexuality, but with navigating two different worldviews of sexuality and family within the relationship. The primary sexual concern was the couple's reluctance to engage in sexual behavior until they resolved their conflicting views. As such, there was no immediate need for psychosexual education. Instead, it was evident that the couple needed to focus on developing cultural appreciation for each other's religious faith traditions, which required religious education as a starting point.

As neither partner was particularly religious, it was important for both of them to gain a deeper understanding of each other's religious backgrounds and their own. To facilitate this process, I asked each partner to reflect on the aspects of their faith that they most appreciated. This involved identifying qualities or principles within their religion that held personal significance, rather than simply listing favorite holidays. Examples included togetherness with family, ancestral heritage, and values such as kindness, family importance, and social responsibility. By encouraging introspection, the exercise helped each partner better appreciate their own faith and gain insight into why their partner's religion was important to them. Additionally, previous research has been conducted, which suggests that learning about and respecting each other's faith traditions can lead to greater understanding and acceptance in the relationship, which in turn can promote relationship satisfaction.

During the following session, I had both Ishaaq and Naomi read their list to their partner. I encouraged the listening partner to actively engage and ask questions. For example, when Naomi stated that she appreciated the idea of a family coming together for *Shabbat* (the Jewish Sabbath), Ishaaq asked her to explain what Shabbat was and why the experience was meaningful to her. Likewise, Naomi asked Ishaaq questions concerning *Hajj* and if he had ever planned to make the pilgrimage. At the end of the session, I asked each patient what they had learned about themselves and about their partner during this exercise. Not surprisingly, they both learned more about their faith tradition and that of their partners. They also gained an understanding of why each one felt aspects of their faith tradition were important to pass down to their child.

As the therapeutic process advanced, it became apparent that the partners needed to deepen their understanding of each other's faiths by experiencing them firsthand. By attending religious services or community events, Ishaaq and Naomi would be able to immerse themselves in the cultural and religious aspects of each other's traditions. In order to get the most out of this experience, I suggested they aim to attend two events each week, one for each partner's religion, and alternate between them. If they were unable to commit to two events, then alternating each week would also suffice. This would allow them to explore their own religious community and identify how they fit in, while also gaining exposure to their partner's community. It was important for Ishaaq and Naomi, both of whom lacked a strong religious background, to broaden their understanding of their respective faiths and the impact they had on their partner. By doing so, they would develop a greater appreciation for their partner's beliefs and strengthen their relationship as they navigated the differences in their worldviews.

Furthermore, it was crucial for the couple to acknowledge the impact of their parents on their relationship and take steps to address any issues that may arise from their involvement. Often, in-law situations can be a source of conflict and tension in a relationship, especially when partners feel that they have to take their parents' side, even if it means going against their partner's wishes or feelings.

To improve the in-law situation, the couple can start by setting clear boundaries with their parents and communicating their needs and expectations effectively (Prentice, 2009). They can also work on building a positive relationship with their in-laws by spending quality time with them, showing appreciation and respect for their traditions and values, and finding common interests to bond over. Further, I suggested that if these tools did not provide a positive outcome, then the entire family may benefit from a family therapist to help navigate any complex family dynamics and improve communication and understanding between all parties involved (Barkham et al., 2021, 539–582).

The conclusion of Ishaaq and Naomi's case was unexpected. Both partners expressed gratitude for the therapy process that allowed them to explore their faith traditions. They gained a greater appreciation for each other's faith and learned a lot about each other. However, they both ultimately concluded that religion was not very important to them. They had only followed their family and tradition due to societal pressure. Nonetheless, they decided to continue living their lives in the same way they had been before Naomi was pregnant and decided that they would raise their child in the same environment. When asked about which holidays and important life cycle events their child would adopt, they responded that they would let the child choose their own path in the future. This suggests that while the couple did not prioritize religion, they still recognized its significance and were open to their child exploring it in the future.

Case Study 3 – Steven and Britney

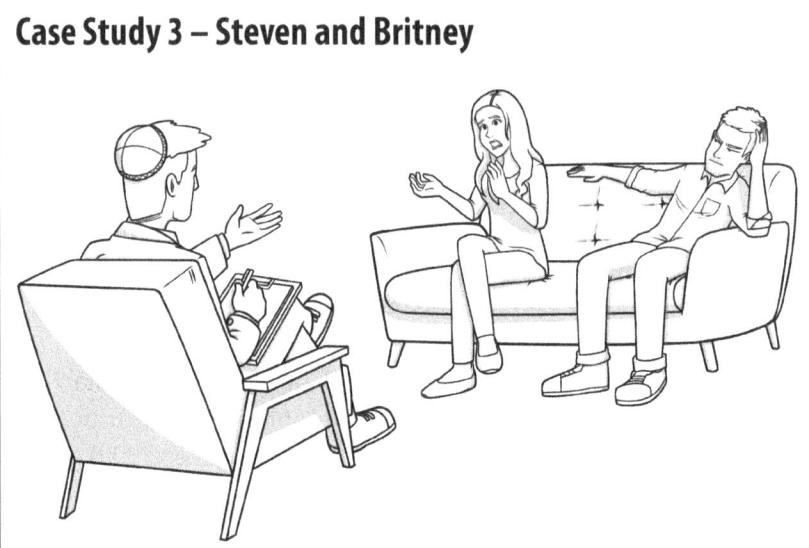

Steven, 31, and Britney, 29, have been married for ten years. They grew up attending the same local church where Britney's father is the pastor. The couple shared that, while they were still children, people have always said that they would end up getting married. Britney describes their wedding as a "dream wedding." However, she feels the relationship has become more of a nightmare since Steven has stopped attending church and says he no longer believes in its teachings.

Steven recalls how he had a question from the Bible that his pastor and other religious leaders couldn't satisfactorily answer. He searched online and found someone on YouTube who addressed the topic. He was surprised and shocked by what he heard, which ultimately caused him to question his faith. This led him to a place of "spiritual turmoil" and he began to study and pray, ultimately concluding that everything he had once believed was a lie. This caused him to leave the church that he grew up in. He says that while he loves Britney, when he looks back he feels he was pushed into marrying her so young. Additionally, he feels lied to by everyone in his life.

Britney is extremely hurt and feels betrayed. She cannot believe that Steven would abandon their faith and is devastated that he would even question their relationship. She states, "I just don't know who he is anymore." During this time, she felt it best that the couple refrain from having sex "until Steven figures his stuff," both spiritually and with regard to their relationship. Steven believes her refusal to have sex is just another form of manipulation that is common within their religious community. Britney says she wants Steven to come back to church and for the couple to continue the life that they had together. She says she has difficulty explaining to their children why their dad is no longer attending church. Steven says that he cannot believe a lie and that Britney should not try to force her beliefs on him if she wishes for the relationship to continue.

Initial Interaction

Upon first meeting Steven, it was clear that he was going through a difficult time. He seemed to be carrying a heavy burden, and his body language and facial expressions conveyed his emotional distress. His eyes were downcast, and his shoulders were hunched, as if he was trying to make himself as small as possible. Steven appeared to be deeply hurt and betrayed by the people he had trusted to guide him spiritually, and this left him feeling disillusioned and lost.

Britney, on the other hand, looked just as troubled, but for different reasons. She seemed scared and confused, unsure of what the future holds for their relationship. It was evident that she was deeply invested in her faith and her church, and Steven's rejection of these things had left her feeling uncertain about their shared future. She kept glancing over at him as if searching for some sign of understanding or connection, but Steven appeared to be lost in his own thoughts.

As they sat together, there was a palpable awkwardness between them, and it was clear that they were struggling to communicate effectively. They seemed to have different goals and motivations for the discussion, with little common ground between them. Steven appeared to be seeking answers and validation for his newfound beliefs, while Britney was hoping to bring him back into the fold of their shared faith. This tension created a barrier between them, making it difficult for them to connect emotionally and find a way forward.

Upon the introduction of the PLISSIT model, an apprehensive silence hung in the room as both partners fixed their gaze upon me. I explicitly requested permission to delve into the realm of sexual topics, recognizing their pivotal relevance to the therapy, yet their response appeared tinged with surprise. Despite the initial hesitancy, they eventually consented, albeit with a hint of reluctance. It was important to address this topic throughout the therapeutic journey, whenever I felt needed within a given situation. Nevertheless, both partners granted permissions to themselves and each other to engage in intimate discussions in the confines of therapy.

Step 1 – Identify

The couple are experiencing an intrareligious conflict. The shared faith and belief system, which once served as the foundation of their relationship, is now causing a rift between them. They both grew up in the same religious community and have always held the same beliefs and worldview. However, Steven's recent rejection of their faith has caused significant turmoil and uncertainty for their future together. As a result, they now find themselves grappling with the challenge of communicating their differing religious views and resolving conflicts that arise due to their contrasting beliefs. This situation can be particularly challenging since the rejection of a shared faith system can bring up deep feelings of disappointment, confusion, and even anger, which can create additional tension in the relationship.

Step 2 – Uncover

The conflict within Steven and Britney's marriage is deeply entwined with their Christian faith and is influenced by several biblical principles. The concept of being "unequally yoked" is rooted in 2 Corinthians 6:14–15 (English Standard Version), which explicitly advises against forming close relationships, including marriage, with unbelievers. Steven's abandonment of his faith can be perceived as a violation of this principle, causing tension within their faith tradition as it challenges the scriptural wisdom of such unions.

Christianity places immense significance on faith as a pathway to salvation and righteous living. Britney's unwavering commitment to her faith, coupled with her fervent desire for Steven to return to the church, underscores the centrality of faith in their lives. Steven's rejection of Christianity is viewed as a profound departure from this core principle, leading to a profound inner conflict within himself and, consequently, within their marriage.

Moreover, the expectations within their family and community exacerbate the conflict. In many Christian communities, there exists a strong expectation that couples share the same faith and actively participate in church life. Given that Britney's father holds a pastoral role, these expectations are likely amplified within her family and community. Steven's departure from the church challenges these communal and familial norms, contributing to the ongoing discord.

The biblical ideal of marital unity is emphasized, encouraging couples to be of one mind and spirit. Steven's spiritual journey away from Christianity disrupts this unity, creating a stark contrast with the biblical vision of a harmonious Christian marriage as detailed in 1 Corinthians 1:10 (English Standard Version). This disconnect generates tension within their relationship as they navigate their diverging paths.

Furthermore, the conflict could extend to their church community, as described in Matthew 18:15–17 (English Standard Version), which provides guidance on resolving conflicts within the church. If their marital struggles become known within their church, it may prompt intervention and concerted efforts to facilitate Steven's return to the faith. This ecclesiastical involvement could exacerbate the conflict further as the couple grapples with external pressures. In line with Ephesians 5:22–33 (English Standard Version), which delineates the roles of husbands and wives in Christian marriage, the husband is traditionally expected to be the spiritual leader of the family. Steven's rejection of his faith challenges this established understanding of marital roles, introducing an additional layer of tension within their relationship.

Finally, the concept of losing one's faith is inherently distressing within Christian theology, as underscored by Hebrews 10:26–27 (English Standard Version). This passage warns against willful sin after gaining knowledge of the truth, suggesting that there is no longer a sacrifice for sins. Steven's inner turmoil and spiritual journey may evoke profound distress and feelings of guilt, further contributing to the conflict within their relationship.

Step 3 – Recognize

When working with Britney and Steven, there are a number of ethical dilemmas that may arise on the part of the clinician. First and foremost the topic of pornography is controversial even within the field of sex therapy, clinicians often have various viewpoints. Therefore, a clinician who has a negative view of pornography, could more easily side with Britney, and could also Influence the treatment direction. This is especially true since many religious clinicians are more likely to hold to concepts of addiction in relation to pornography.

Step 4 – Develop

Going into this therapeutic partnership, I wanted to establish the motivation for each partner to put in the work in order to make the marriage last. For this particular couple, I decided not to incorporate their faith tradition, not only because Steven had left the faith, but also because Britney's scriptural influence to remain married, is based upon an ulterior motive – belief that Steven would come back to church. Thus, I wanted the couple to search for motivation, based upon characteristics that they valued in their partner and aspects of their relationship that they treasure and appreciate.

Both partners were able to come up with a list of personal characteristics and relationship aspects that were meaningful to them. It was noticeable, while each partner shared their list in therapy, that their words were deeply meaningful to their partner. It was then I recognized that despite Steven's hesitation toward the relationship, he did in fact love Britney very much, and her feelings toward him had never altered. In order to move forward, I suggested reframing their relationship narrative without the religious components. For the following weeks, we focused on remembering the early stages of their relationship, emphasizing their individual connection rather than their shared religious experience. For example, Steven initially shared his first encounter with Britney as follows:

> "We went to the same church, she was always there because her father was the pastor. I immediately had a crush on her and people always commented how I would marry the pastor's daughter one day."

He later reframed the experience without the religious component as follows:

> "I remember seeing this girl with a ribbon in her hair and thinking she had pretty eyes. I was like nine or ten so all my friends would tease me for having a crush on her. I never managed to get the courage to ask her out until I was like fifteen, I had never dated any other girls because I always hoped someday Britney would like me."

Reframing the narrative was crucial as it enabled the patient to refocus on the emotions he had towards his partner during the early stages of their relationship. This allowed him to see that the religious aspect, which he currently rejects, did not have as significant an impact on the fate of their relationship as he initially thought. As a result, he was able to accept their relationship. Through this process, Britney realized that Steven's rejection of their shared faith was not a rejection of her, but rather a personal decision. Over the course of six weeks, the couple were given homework assignments to reframe significant moments of their relationship including special memories while dating, their engagement, their wedding, and the birth of their children. These exercises helped both partners to acknowledge and appreciate their relationship for what it is, despite their differing beliefs.

While this part of the therapeutic journey was successful in excavating the foundations upon which their relationship was based, there were still some problematic issues that needed to be resolved, including Britney's concern over Steven's influence on their children's spirituality. This became an area of significant dispute. I quickly became thankful that the couple had recently discovered their deep love for one another, because while discussing the fate of their children's upbringing, it was clear that their relationship could have quickly crumbled. Steven expressed that he could not bring himself to deceive his children and allow them to follow a religion he now deemed false. On the other hand, Britney strongly desired to raise their children in the same church she had grown up in. To add to the complexity of the situation, Britney's father was not only the pastor of the church but also Steven's father-in-law and the grandfather to their children. This family dynamic only made it more challenging for the couple to navigate this issue.

Moving forward, I decided to help the couple first establish boundaries with their in-laws, primarily Britney's father. Both described her father as a very caring and loving man, however, due to his religious convictions, he was involving himself more than usual in their relationship since Steven's decision to leave the church. To begin with, I worked with the couple to identify specific areas where Britney's father had been overstepping their boundaries. Steven expressed that he felt that Britney's father was trying to influence their decisions as a couple, particularly when it came to their children's religious upbringing. Britney, on the other hand, felt that her father was simply trying to be helpful and did not see it as an issue.

Together, we came up with two concrete ways that the couple could establish boundaries with Britney's father. First, they decided to limit the amount of time that they spent with him, especially when discussing topics related to religion. This allowed them to have more control over the conversations that they had with him and prevented him from becoming too involved in their relationship. Second, they decided to be more assertive in their communication with him, clearly expressing their opinions and desires when it came to their children's religious upbringing. With these boundaries in place, the couple found that they were better able to navigate their relationship with Britney's father and reduce the conflict that had been causing tension in their marriage.

Next, it was important to address the issue of the religious upbringing of their child. It was apparent that the couple needed to find ways to compromise. I offered the couple three options for doing this. First, they could try a "both-and" approach, whereby the couple could try to find ways to incorporate both partners' beliefs and values into their child's upbringing. Second, they could choose to wait until the child was older and could make an informed decision themselves on their religious belief system. Lastly, I suggested that the couple could simply agree to disagree. It is important to recognize that sometimes it is not possible to reach a compromise but they can still support each other as parents and focus on teaching their child important values and principles that are important to both of them, such as kindness, respect, and empathy.

After more than a year of therapy, Steven and Britney have demonstrated remarkable progress in their marriage. Throughout the course of their therapy, they have gained important communication skills that have enabled them to address and navigate day-to-day issues with greater ease. They have established clear boundaries, which have helped them to establish a sense of stability in their relationship. While they have made considerable progress, they still occasionally quarrel over the religious upbringing of their children.

This issue tends to surface more frequently during religious holidays and other religious events, which they both describe as being particularly challenging moments. Nevertheless, despite these ongoing struggles, the couple has demonstrated extreme resilience and commitment toward one another. They have expressed a deep desire to continue working on their marriage and to continuously strive to improve the relationship that they share.

Through therapy, Steven and Britney have been able to develop a deeper understanding and appreciation for one another. They have come to see that their differing beliefs do not have to be a source of conflict in their marriage. Instead, they have learned to value and respect each other's beliefs and to find ways to celebrate their differences. This has enabled them to build a stronger foundation of trust and mutual respect, which has helped them to navigate the challenges that they face as a couple.

In conclusion, while Steven and Britney's marriage has not been without its challenges, they have demonstrated a willingness to work through their issues and to commit to one another. They have shown that with hard work and dedication, it is possible to build a strong and enduring marriage, even when faced with significant differences in beliefs and values.

Conclusion

Working with interfaith and intrafaith couples in sex therapy requires therapists to have an understanding of the different cultural and religious beliefs that can influence a couple's sexual health and satisfaction. This chapter has shown that communication is essential for addressing the challenges faced by these couples. By helping couples to acknowledge their differences, identify their values and beliefs, and find ways to incorporate them into their sexual expression, therapists can provide meaningful support to improve their sexual and relational well-being.

The three case examples presented in this chapter demonstrate the importance of a culturally sensitive approach when working with interfaith and intrafaith couples in sex therapy. In each case, the couples faced different challenges related to their religious and cultural backgrounds. However, through therapy, they were able to gain a deeper understanding of each other's perspectives and develop stronger communication skills to address their issues.

Overall, it is crucial for therapists to approach interfaith and intrafaith couples in sex therapy with an open mind and a non-judgmental attitude. By acknowledging and respecting the diversity of their patients' religious and cultural backgrounds, therapists can provide effective and meaningful support to improve their sexual and relational well-being. It is important to recognize that each couple's experiences are unique and may require a tailored approach to therapy. By providing a safe and accepting space for couples to explore their sexual and relational issues, therapists can help them navigate the challenges and find new ways to connect and grow together.

Note

1 It is also possible to have a person of faith married to an atheist. While it is perhaps obvious the conflicts that this dynamic could cause within the relationship itself, it could also cause problems within the microsystem of the couple. In a 2014 Pew Study, 77% of evangelicals said they would be unhappy if their family member married an atheist (Lipka & Martínez, 2014).

References

Barkham, M., Lutz, W., & Castonguay, L. G. (Eds.). (2021). *Bergin and Garfield's Handbook of Psychotherapy and Behavior Change.* Wiley.

Baskin, J. R. (Ed.). (1998). *Jewish Women in Historical Perspective.* Wayne State University Press.

Cerchiaro, F. (2020). Identity loss or identity re-shape? Religious identification among the offspring of "Christian–Muslim" couples. *Journal of Contemporary Religion, 35*(3), 503–521. DOI: 10.1080/13537903.2020.1839250

Lehman, M., Kanarek, J. L., & Bronner, S. J. (Eds.). (2017). *Mothers in the Jewish Cultural Imagination: Jewish Cultural Studies*, volume 5. Liverpool University Press.

Lipka, M., & Martínez, J. (2014). So, you married an atheist … Retrieved from http://pewrsr.ch/1uy4Z7t

Prentice, C. (2009). Relational dialectics among in-laws. *Journal of Family Communication, 9*(2), 67–89. DOI: 10.1080/15267430802561667

Ramadan, T. (2017). *Introduction to Islam* (F. A. Reed, Trans.). Oxford University Press.

11

Nonmonogamy

Introduction

In recent years, the discourse surrounding non-monogamous relationship structures has significantly expanded, capturing increasing attention and recognition within both the specialized field of sex therapy and the broader landscape of popular culture (Braida et al., 2023). However, it is necessary to acknowledge that the concept of non-monogamy is far from novel, as it has been an integral part of diverse cultures worldwide throughout the annals of history (Watson & Stein Lubrano, 2021). Within this multifaceted domain, two primary paradigms of non-monogamy emerge as noteworthy: **polygamy** and **polyamory**, each possessing its unique dynamics and complexities (Füllgrabe & Smith, 2023).

Polygamy is a marital arrangement wherein an individual is simultaneously involved in multiple spousal relationships simultaneously (Krenawi, 2012). This practice diverges from monogamy, where a person is exclusively committed to one spouse. Three distinct subcategories emerge within polygamy, each characterized by unique relationship dynamics. **Polygyny** involves a man being married to multiple wives concurrently (Matsumura, 2022). This form of polygamy has historical and cultural roots in various societies worldwide. In polygynous unions, the husband maintains multiple distinct marital relationships, and each wife may or may not have direct relationships with one

DOI: 10.4324/9781003242017-15

another. The dynamics within polygyny can be complex, often necessitating open and transparent communication to navigate issues of fairness, intimacy, and familial responsibilities.

In contrast, **polyandry**, a marriage arrangement where a woman has multiple husbands simultaneously, is a less common but documented practice in certain societies (Fjeld, 2022). It has been observed in regions such as Nepal, parts of India, and remote areas of China. Finally, **polygynandry**, a relatively lesser-known variant of polygamy, has been observed in regions such as Tibet, Nepal, and Bhutan. It encompasses the practice of multiple men and women engaging in simultaneous relationships within a collective group dynamic. Within these arrangements, individuals have the opportunity to form romantic or sexual connections with multiple partners, and all members of the group may potentially engage in interconnected relationships. This form of polygamy introduces a multifaceted interplay of emotions, shared responsibilities, and power dynamics, highlighting the importance of fostering open communication and cultivating mutual understanding among all parties involved.

The other prevalent form of non-monogamous relationships, gaining popularity, particularly within sex therapy, is **polyamory**. Often used interchangeably with ethical non-monogamy or consensual non-monogamy, polyamory allows individuals to engage in multiple romantic or sexual relationships, all with the informed knowledge and consent of everyone involved (Domínguez et al., 2017). Prominent publications like *The Ethical Slut* and *More Than Two* have significantly contributed to the discourse surrounding ethical non-monogamy, placing a strong emphasis on principles such as transparent communication, unwavering honesty, and the cultivation of mutual respect among partners (Hardy & Easton, 2017; Veaux et al., 2014). Clinicians must recognize the profound significance of making informed and ethical choices within the intricate domain of love and desire, particularly in polyamorous relationships.

The concept of non-monogamy is far from novel, with historical instances documented across various cultures. Among the Abrahamic Faith Traditions, both Judaism and Islam, depending on the cultural context, have historically allowed polygamy at different times. Christianity, in contrast, has consistently opposed the practice. Nevertheless, all three faith traditions strongly emphasize the sanctity of sex within the bounds of marriage. As such, non-monogamous relationships can present significant challenges for religious individuals seeking to align their beliefs with their intimate relationships. Navigating these complexities requires a sensitive and nuanced approach from clinicians, who must be attuned to the unique intersection of faith, intimacy, and personal values in the lives of their religious patients.

Therapist Bias Check

1. Am I respecting the patient's religiously informed desire to stay monogamous?
2. Do I have negative attitudes toward polygamy?

Case Study 1 – Tovia and Yael

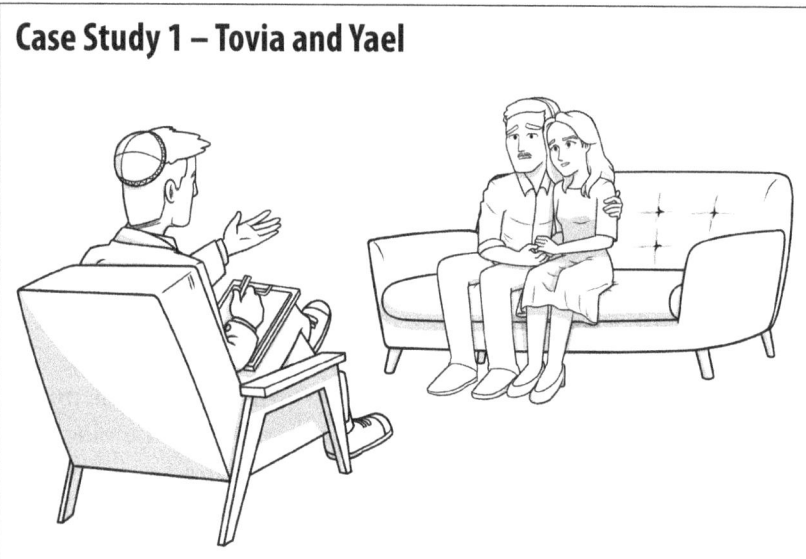

Tovia (23) and Yael (23) were recently thrown out of their Yeshiva, where they were studying for the Rabbinate. They had been involved with the program for some time and were actively teaching when the incident happened. Several people involved in the Yeshiva were part of an orgy in which Yael took part. Tovia, who says he and his wife were involved in poly-amorous relationships, was unaware she participated in this particular orgy. One of the female participants later commented to one of the directors of the Yeshiva that she was impressed that the Yeshiva was progressive and "forward thinking" and that they allowed staff to be involved in non-monogamous relationships. This led to Tovia and Yael being called to the office to have a discussion with the leadership of the program. Despite Yael telling them that Tovia did not know she had taken part in the orgy, they were both forced to leave the program since they openly practiced polyamory. Now, both partners feel they have no sense of direction and purpose, and Tovia blames Yael for ruining his future.

Initial Interaction

Upon the commencement of Tovia and Yael's initial appointment, a palpable sense of nervousness and trepidation enveloped the room, unsurprising given their recent expulsion from Rabbinical school, a source of profound hurt and devastation. To establish a foundation of comfort and trust, I initiated the session by outlining our objectives and introduced the critical permission component of the PLISSIT model. In recognizing the potential discomfort surrounding discussions of sexuality, I candidly requested their consent to delve into sexual matters. I explained that as someone who talks about sex all the time, I sometimes forget it can be uncomfortable for others, so I wanted to ask their permission to discuss sex with them. Their shared, albeit slightly amused, agreement served as an initial breakthrough, granting them the reassurance of their agency in shaping the therapeutic journey ahead.

As our conversations unfolded, it became evident that Yael was hesitant to acknowledge her role in the relationship strain and appeared emotionally distant from Tovia, casting doubt on her commitment to their shared future. Conversely, Tovia's responses oscillated between assigning blame to Yael and critiquing the Yeshiva and Orthodox Judaism as overarching culprits in their predicament. These interactions unveiled a complex internal conflict within Tovia, one entangled with his religious convictions. Yet, the underlying motives behind this turmoil remained unclear, leaving us to question whether it stemmed from personal trauma or his pursuit of holding the religious system accountable for his profound disappointment.

Step 1 – Identify

Both members of the couple were raised in devoutly religious households and felt a strong calling towards the Rabbinate. However, their polyamorous lifestyle led to the opportunity being revoked. Moreover, there appears to be a disagreement between Tovia and Yael regarding the boundaries of their polyamorous arrangement. This indicates either a lack of communication between them about their relationship's parameters or one partner's reluctance to honor and adhere to their agreement.

Step 2 – Uncover

Since the time of Gershom ben Judah, Judaism has adopted monogamy as the only standard for the family (Jacobson & Hirt, 2021). This commitment to monogamy is deeply rooted in Biblical and Talmudic texts. In the Hebrew Bible, Genesis 2:24 emphasizes the union of one man and one woman in marriage, stating, "Therefore a man shall leave his father and his mother and hold fast to his wife, and they shall become one flesh." The Seventh Commandment, "You shall not commit adultery" (Exodus 20:14), further underscores the importance of marital fidelity. These biblical teachings lay the foundation for the traditional Jewish view of marriage as a sacred covenant between one man and one woman, marked by exclusivity and faithfulness.

The Talmud, a central text in Rabbinic Judaism, expands on these principles. It contains extensive discussions on marital fidelity and prohibited sexual relationships. For instance, in the Babylonian Talmud, tractate Sanhedrin 76b, it is discussed that the Talmudic sage Rava ruled that a polygamous marriage contract was invalid, reflecting the prevailing interpretation of monogamy in Rabbinic Judaism. Additionally, the Talmudic tractate Yevamot explores the laws related to marriage, demonstrating the Talmud's emphasis on monogamy and the prohibition of extramarital sexual relations. Orthodox Judaism holds these teachings dear, viewing marriage as a holy union that demands the utmost commitment and loyalty. Consequently, the pursuit of polyamorous relationships, as seen in the case of Tovia and Yael, is considered inconsistent with Orthodox Jewish beliefs and practices, leading to their expulsion from the Yeshiva and raising significant moral and religious questions within the community.

Step 3 – Recognize

Several ethical dilemmas may surface when working with a situation similar to that of Tovia and Yael. For therapists who prioritize polyamory-friendly perspectives, potential discord may arise due to conflicts with the couple's religious convictions regarding monogamy. This scenario could lead clinicians to exhibit unconscious sympathies or biases, inadvertently favoring one partner over the other. Which could also arise if it is viewed that one partner is suffering the consequences of his partners actions. Furthermore, religious therapists might harbor preconceived notions that a religious couple, particularly one involving a future rabbi, would lean towards an unconventional relationship style, further complicating the ethical terrain.

Step 4 – Develop

Throughout the therapeutic process with this couple, it became increasingly evident that the available avenues for facilitating their return to rabbinical school were quite constrained. A potential course of action suggested was the exploration of alternative, more liberal rabbinical programs that might have been more accommodating to their unique circumstances. Nevertheless, it became evident that neither party displayed a particular inclination towards pursuing their education at a non-Orthodox training institution, as their unwavering commitment to Orthodox Judaism remained paramount.

The primary individual grappling with the complexities of their situation was Tovia. He found himself wrestling not only with the challenges to his faith but also with the strains on his relationship with Yael. On one hand, he harbored resentment towards the school for their expulsion, seeing it as an unjust decision. Simultaneously, he held Yael accountable for the circumstances that led to their expulsion, contributing to a palp-able inner conflict. Tovia's emotional state was characterized by turmoil, and he frequently expressed thoughts of renouncing his Judaism and even contemplated severing his relationship with Yael. These discussions underscored the deep emotional conflicts he was experiencing and highlighted the need for therapeutic support to navigate the intricate interplay between his faith and his relationship.

Considering the importance of integrating a patient's reli-gious beliefs into therapy, it is often encouraged for patients to explore their spiritual interests and growth. However, it is essen-tial to recognize that most therapists, unless they have received formal theological training, may not have the expertise required to effectively support patients on their spiritual journeys. In other words, therapists without theological training or clerical affiliations should exercise caution when providing spiritual guidance within a therapeutic context. This is akin to a member of the clergy attempting to deliver intensive trauma therapy without the necessary training and skills. In such situations, seeking consultation with a qualified member of the clergy is advisable.

Nevertheless, within the context of this particular scenario, it became evident that a more in-depth exploration of the dynamics within the partnered relationship was warranted. It became apparent that certain boundary-related challenges had arisen within the framework of their consensual non-monogamous arrangement. Consequently, a conversation was initiated with the couple, inviting them to share insights into the motivations behind their choice of this relationship style.

Yael expressed a desire for sexual involvement with individ-uals outside of their partnership as her motivation for wanting a non-monogamous relationship agreement. Tovia not only wanted to make his partner happy but also identified as having a more contemporary and open perspective and acquiesced to relationship styles. However, it became apparent that the depth of their discussion on the matter was somewhat limited, leaving room for a more comprehensive examination of their consensual non-monogamous dynamics.

This led to **psychosexual education** regarding consensual non-monogamy. It was primarily stressing the importance of negotiations between the couple and the importance of setting boundaries. It became more apparent during these discussions that the couple had not previously communicated much beyond the agreement to be polygamous. Jael, however, did not seem to think it was of much importance and felt that her non-monogamy should be spontaneous whenever she chose or felt sexual desire toward another person. By his response, it was clear that Tovia was totally uncomfortable with this suggestion.

Tovia shared a story in which Jael had invited a partner over for a morning encounter just before he departed for work. He mentioned that as he left for work, he could hear Jael and this other partner engaging in sexual activity. Upon returning home, he found them still involved in such activity. Tovia acknowledged that this experience deeply affected him, and he frequently returned from work with anxiety about potentially hearing Jael with other individuals.

Recognizing the apparent need for intervention in the couple's relationship dynamics, an opportune moment arose to **incorporate their faith tradition** into the therapeutic process. Centering discussions around the significance of marriage in Judaism, both partners responded with resistance. Tovia, not-ably, displayed heightened emotional reactions, deeply affected by his faith tradition's perspective on marriage, albeit in a distressing manner. Conversely, Jael's response remained rela-tively indifferent, as if the topic held little relevance. In light of these reactions, a strategic shift was made. Instead of directly addressing the theological aspects, the focus transitioned to a more introspective inquiry. Each partner was invited to share their personal reflections on their marriage, fostering a deeper exploration of their individual perspectives and emotional reactions.

Tovia openly conveyed his profound affection for his partner and his aspiration to build a life characterized by mutual support. In contrast, while acknowledging her care for Tovia, Jael revealed that marriage did not hold a particularly high priority for her. She candidly shared that her consideration of marriage might have been different had she not grown up within the Jewish context. This revelation triggered further discussions regarding the trajectory of their relationship.

During these conversations, Jael openly acknowledged her spontaneous approach to life and her outlook on the relationship's future. This revelation underscored a noteworthy disparity in perspective between the two partners, shedding light on the challenges that permeated their relationship.

Regrettably, at this juncture in our therapeutic journey, the discussions brought both partners' conflicts within their marriage into sharper focus, rendering the search for **creative solutions** a formidable task. Tovia found himself grappling with emotional distress, and it appeared that Jael's level of empathy fell short of his needs. Consequently, taking a direct approach allowed a candid question to be asked of the couple, inquiring about their desires for their relationship. Uncertainty prevailed in their responses, but Jael articulated a sentiment: "Whatever happens, I hope that Tovia and I can always remain friends." This statement prompted my subsequent question: "Does this mean that you would be open to the idea of a get (a Jewish document of divorce)?" Both partners responded affirmatively to this query with a shared "yes."

Not ready to give up on the couple just yet, a joint homework assignment was assigned, where each partner was tasked with composing a list outlining what they believed would be essential for the relationship to succeed. Crucially, this task was to be carried out independently, without any discussion or sharing between them outside the therapy room. During the subsequent session, both partners presented their respective lists.

As each partner's list unfolded, it became increasingly evident that their core values and relationship expectations were not aligned. Jael expressed a desire for Tovia to embrace her spontaneous approach to non-monogamy, whereas Tovia sought greater consistency and stability within their relationship.

After an intensive five and a half months of therapy, the couple ultimately arrived at the painful decision to bring their relationship to a close. In this particular case, finding a compromise that satisfied both partners proved an insurmountable challenge. Additionally, it became clear that Tovia carried deep emotional wounds resulting from past actions by Jael, for which she did not take full responsibility. Fortunately, within the framework of Judaism, divorce is a permissible option, and neither partner voiced objections to pursuing this course of action. The couple continued to engage in therapy for an additional month, navigating the intricate terrain of their divorce proceedings.

Case Study 2 – Jackson and Taylor

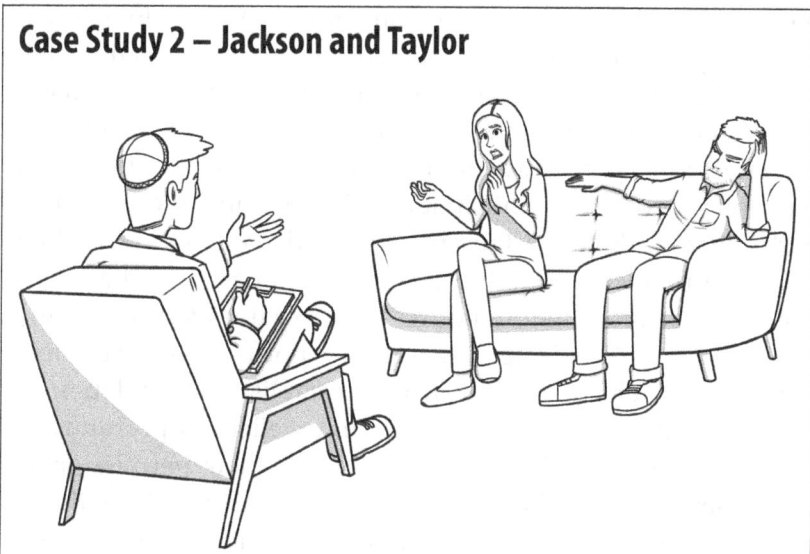

Jackson (26) and Taylor (22) have been married for just a year. Taylor has a son named Tommy (5) from pregnancy during high school, long before she met Jackson. During her pregnancy with Tommy, Taylor began attending a local Apostolic Pentecostal Church, where she eventually crossed paths with Jackson. Presently, both remain actively engaged in their church, with each holding leadership roles in various programs. Recently, a situation unfolded within their congregation when the pastor became aware of several couples engaging in group sexual activities. In response, the pastor implemented a new guideline restricting married couples to meeting only in public settings. Jackson and Taylor have confessed to participating in such encounters with other couples and continue to do so. They are anxious that the pastor may discover their involvement and subsequently exclude them from the ministries they are actively engaged in. Additionally, Taylor is grappling with nightmares that her son, Tommy, may eventually distance himself from the church due to her past actions, which she perceives as "transgressions."

Initial Interaction

In the course of their clinical session, Jackson and Taylor exuded a vibrant, youthful enthusiasm toward life and their relationship. Within the initial moments of our dialogue, Taylor's remark, "I can't believe I am actually meeting with a sex therapist," resonated not with shock or resentment but with a profound sense of wonder and anticipation. Recognizing the prevalent myths surrounding sex therapy, I probed their understanding and uncertainties about the practice, emphasizing that their consent was paramount in addressing sexual issues despite my professional role. This approach aimed not only to dispel any lingering apprehensions but also to establish a foundation of trust and comfort. It also served as an excellent opportunity to introduce the PLISSIT model and ask for their permission to discuss sexual issues. Likewise, I requested that they give themselves permission to discuss sex in our session assuring them it was a private and confidential environment.

It became apparent that both harbored a certain cognitive innocence, reflected in their conservative attire, somewhat unconventional for the season. Throughout our session, their palpable nervousness underscored the discomfort associated with discussing personal matters in a therapeutic context, prompting me to consistently seek their consent and reassure them of their agency. Eventually, Jackson and Taylor bravely disclosed their premarital sexual activity, something that they had never shared before, which undoubtedly seemed to amplify their distorted thought patterns and emotional turmoil. Despite these challenges, their unwavering commitment to nurturing a thriving marriage deeply rooted in their Apostolic Pentecostal beliefs remained evident, underscoring their determination to align their faith tradition with their aspirations for a harmonious family life.

Step 1 – Identify

The couple initially sought therapy because they decided to open their relationship with another couple from their church. However, it quickly became evident that several underlying factors contributed to their situation. They disclosed that they had engaged in sexual activity before marriage, which had led them to marry hastily due to the guilt and shame associated with their premarital behavior.

Furthermore, the couple explained that their involvement in group sexual activities with another couple from their church had initially added excitement and enjoyment to their relationship. Nevertheless, they also acknowledged experiencing overwhelming guilt and fear, which were beginning to have an adverse impact on their relationship with each other and their spiritual connection.

Taylor expressed deep concern about the possibility that the other couple might reveal their activities to someone in the church or their pastor, foreseeing potential complications. The revelation that their pastor had already learned about some couples in the church engaging in open relationships was the final straw that made the burden of secrecy too challenging for the couple to bear alone.

The couple candidly expressed a shared belief that their current lifestyle choices could lead them to eternal damnation. This deep-seated fear about the fate of their souls weighed heavily on both of them. Moreover, they were profoundly concerned about the potential impact of their present choices on the spiritual well-being of their child, Tommy. Both partners disclosed that they grappled with what they described as a sexual addiction, which left them feeling powerless to control their impulses. This acknowledgment underscored the urgency of addressing their emotional and psychological challenges within the therapeutic context.

Step 2 – Uncover

According to Fundamentalist Christian teachings derived from the Christian Bible, Jackson and Taylor's situation contradicts their faith's teachings on several fronts. Premarital and extramarital sex are considered sinful within these teachings. The Christian Bible includes various passages emphasizing the sanctity of marriage and the importance of sexual purity. For instance, Hebrews 13:4 (English Standard Version) states, "Let marriage be held in honor among all, and let the marriage bed be undefiled, for God will judge the sexually immoral and adulterous." The Christian ideal of monogamy is upheld in passages like Genesis 2:24 (English Standard Version): "Therefore a man shall leave his father and his mother and hold fast to his wife, and they shall become one flesh." Engaging in group sexual activities or polyamorous relationships stands in direct contrast to this monogamous standard.

Moreover, Christian teachings strongly condemn adultery, which includes extramarital sexual relations. The Seventh Commandment, "You shall not commit adultery" (Exodus 20:14, English Standard Version), is a cornerstone of Christian ethics. Participation in sexual activities with multiple partners, other than one's spouse, is regarded as a breach of this commandment. While Christian doctrine emphasizes the possibility of forgiveness through repentance and faith in Jesus Christ, continuous involvement in behavior contrary to biblical principles may lead to spiritual turmoil and a sense of alienation from God.

Lastly, many Christian denominations have specific conduct standards for their members, especially those in leadership roles. Engaging in behavior conflicting with these standards, such as participating in group sexual activities, may result in disciplinary measures within the church community. In essence, Jackson and Taylor's situation is at odds with their faith due to premarital and extramarital sexual activities, deviation from monogamous principles, violation of biblical commandments related to sexual purity and marital fidelity, and the potential disruption of their standing within their faith community and relationship with God.

Step 3 – Recognize

In the case of Jackson and Taylor, certain therapists may contend that their religion and associated beliefs contribute unwarranted guilt and shame to their sexual decisions, potentially exacerbating a distressingly negative view of their choices. Furthermore, there may be therapists who struggle with disapproval regarding Jackson and Taylor's unwavering commitment to their religious belief system, despite its perceived association with negative attitudes toward sex. In the context of religious therapists, concerns might arise regarding Taylor and Jackson's admission of sexual encounters occurring outside the confines of their marital relationship. These underlying dynamics have the potential to manifest within the therapeutic relationship, potentially straining the therapeutic alliance and impeding patient progress.

Step 4 – Develop

When working with religious patients, the focal point of the approach centers on facilitating the attainment of harmony between their religious beliefs and their sexual practices. This undertaking assumes heightened significance when individuals grapple with the specter of "eternal damnation" resulting from the perceived incongruence between their sexual behaviors and religious convictions. In most instances, suggesting a departure from their faith tradition can intensify these emotional struggles and should, therefore, generally be avoided.

In the case of Jackson and Taylor, the process was initiated by posing a fundamental question: "What are your sexual values?" Frequently, individuals have not engaged in the process of articulating their sexual values or delving into the underlying motivations. Emphasis is placed on steering clear of an examination of church teachings or parental influences from their upbringing. Instead, the focus remains on discerning their intrinsic values concerning sexuality. This initiates a reflective journey that many have not embarked upon previously, offering a valuable avenue for psychosexual education.

A standard practice in couples therapy entails assigning both partners the task of independently compiling an exhaustive catalog of their respective sexual values. This assignment serves as a catalyst for cultivating a more profound comprehension of their individual viewpoints regarding sexuality. During our subsequent session, an in-depth exploration of these values ensues, with an emphasis on prompting each partner to articulate not only the essence of their values but also the underlying reasons that imbue these values with personal significance.

This exercise is a pivotal opportunity for the partners to enrich their understanding of one another's beliefs and attitudes concerning sexuality. Frequently, it unveils not only shared values but also areas of disparity, which have the potential to evolve into future sources of conflict within their relationship. Through proactively exploring these dimensions, couples can forge a pathway towards a more sophisticated comprehension of each other's sexual values. This, in turn, facilitates the construction of a robust foundation characterized by mutual respect and profound understanding in their partnership.

In the subsequent phases of therapy, we delve deeper into the process of helping the partners identify any discrepancies between their personal and religious values concerning sex. This is one way to **incorporate their faith tradition** into the therapeutic process. This step is vital as it enables couples to recognize and acknowledge these differences, setting the stage for potential conflict resolution. In the case of Jackson and Taylor, it became evident that their respective stances on sexuality had not been thoroughly examined.

Within the context of their relationship, Taylor assumed a more assertive role in matters of sexuality, taking the lead in their sexual decisions. In contrast, Jackson had not previously engaged in deep introspection regarding his own sexual values. He tended to defer to Taylor's preferences regarding matters of intimacy. Both partners had not invested substantial time exploring the alignment or divergence between their personal sexual values and their partner's values, and they had yet to consider how these values aligned or conflicted with the teachings of their faith.

Through this exploration, Taylor came to realize that her personal values were more closely aligned with her religious values than she had initially believed. She shared that growing up in a single-parent household marked by her parents' early divorce and her father's incarceration for sexual offenses during her early teens had profoundly influenced her desire for a solid and stable family life. While she expressed that she did not inherently view premarital sex as wrong if it occurred within the context of love, she placed great emphasis on monogamy within a marital relationship. Thus, now, there is a conflict between her personal sexual values and her sexual behavior. This conflict was only enforced by her religion's teachings on extramarital sex.

To help resolve the conflict, the process involves assisting the couple in determining the appropriate sexual boundaries to safeguard their individual sexual values. Emphasis is placed on these boundaries, serving as protective measures, ensuring the well-being of themselves and those around them. One creative approach often employed in this exercise is the encouragement of religiously informed boundaries, which allows individuals to navigate potential discomfort when asserting their desire to uphold specific sexual limits. Essentially, their faith tradition serves as a potent explanatory tool for elucidating to others the rationale behind their chosen sexual boundaries. This approach cultivates a sense of alignment between personal values and religious beliefs, ultimately facilitating a more seamless integration of faith and sexuality.

These boundaries assume a critical role, particularly when navigating interactions with the other couple they had previously engaged in sexual activity. Jackson and Taylor articulated two primary concerns concerning their relationship with this couple. Firstly, they grappled with how to avert further sexual involvement, and secondarily, they harbored apprehensions that the other couple might react negatively and potentially disclose their previous interactions to others.

Addressing their initial concern necessitated a two-pronged strategy. Initially, engaging in a direct conversation with the other couple was essential, articulating their desire to discontinue any sexual involvement. Subsequently, mechanisms needed to be devised to ensure the maintenance of this boundary. To initiate this process, an assignment was issued: composing a letter addressed to the other couple. This letter conveyed their appreciation for the friendship while firmly stating their decision to cease engaging in sexual activities. Importantly, the purpose of this exercise was not to share the letter with the other couple but rather to facilitate the development of effective communication skills. By reading the letter aloud during therapy sessions, Jackson and Taylor could rehearse and refine the words they would later employ in their forthcoming discussion with the other couple.

Within our therapeutic framework aimed at boundary maintenance, we embark on a collaborative journey to establish clear parameters designed to fortify these boundaries. Recognizing that boundaries may sometimes be susceptible to compromise, particularly in the context of sexual desire and familiarity, we adopt a comprehensive approach that encompasses the exploration of positive alternatives.

For instance, Taylor identified a boundary by suggesting that it might be best for them not to spend time alone with the other couple in their respective homes. This serves as an example of a parameter she has set to uphold her boundary. However, to bolster the effectiveness of this boundary, we also explore positive alternatives. These alternatives could include engaging in public activities such as mini-golf, bowling, or sharing a meal together at a restaurant, any activity that is enjoyed by all involved. By incorporating these positive alternatives, we create a proactive strategy that ensures the parameters are maintained and reinforces the initial boundary, reducing the likelihood of boundary violations in situations where sexual attraction and familiarity may pose challenges.

Over time, Jackson and Taylor managed to initiate a candid conversation with their friends, who had likewise struggled to find an appropriate way to broach the topic. This dialogue brought about a profound sense of relief for both partners, as it not only facilitated an understanding between them but also assured Jackson and Taylor that their friends respected their confidentiality regarding their sexual activities with others. Subsequently, the couple has successfully upheld healthy sexual boundaries with their friends, transforming the relationship into something more profound and meaningful. Furthermore, Jackson and Taylor have reported a remarkable resolution of the distress stemming from their fear of eternal damnation. They attribute this transformation to the reconciliation they have achieved between their deeply held personal values and their religious beliefs. This journey has not only strengthened their bond as a couple but has also fortified their connection to their faith in a profoundly transformative way.

Case Study 3 – Hamid

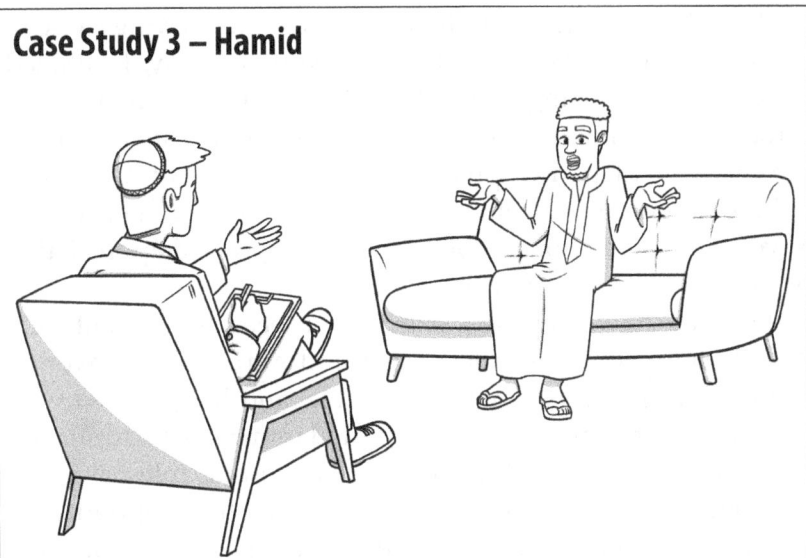

Hamid, a 32-year-old Muslim man originally from Ghana, has been residing in Europe for the past five years. He recently expressed significant challenges related to the cultural differences he has encountered, and he perceives these differences as negatively affecting his family's well-being. Hamid hails from a cultural background where it is not uncommon for Muslim men to have multiple wives. Currently, he is married to two women, Samira (29) and Sherifa (27). Hamid disclosed that he shares two children with Samira, aged 7 and 4, and one child, aged 3, with Sherifa, who is currently pregnant with another child. He deeply desires to be with Sherifa during her pregnancy, but governmental regulations in Europe do not recognize multiple marriages, which has led to immense distress for him. The separation from Sherifa has caused Hamid significant emotional turmoil as he longs for the unity of his family under one roof. He emphasized that the physical distance between his wives and children has led to feelings of severe depression and hopelessness.

Initial Interaction

In my initial meeting with Hamid, he presented as a remarkably gentle and composed individual, though an underlying sense of profound weight was unmistakable. Without delay, I initiated our session, expressing gratitude for his willingness to meet and introduce the PLISSIT model. Seeking his permission to delve into sexual matters, I emphasized the importance of his agency in this dialogue and encouraged him to grant himself permission as well. Hamid graciously consented and expressed appreciation for my considerate approach.

Beneath his composed exterior, it became evident that Hamid harbored deep-seated anger and hurt. His unwavering commitment to his family was palpable, and he grappled with the emotional turmoil of being separated from Sharifa during her pregnancy. He believed that he was failing in his roles as a husband and father by not providing Sharifa with the opportunity to reside with him. This inner conflict ignited his anger, directed both inwardly and toward governmental policies that failed to recognize his plural marriages.

Step 1 – Identify

Hamid's profound struggle to be apart from his second wife, Sherifa, during her pregnancy is deeply entwined with his cultural and religious convictions, which emphasize the significance of unity and familial support. His anguish is intensified by the legal and societal complexities he faces in Europe, where polygamous marriages are not legally recognized. This predicament forces him to navigate the intricate balance between his profound religious convictions and the legal constraints of his current milieu. The inner conflict between his aspiration to fulfill his religious obligations as a husband, as guided by the Quran, and the legal restrictions that impede him from doing so has left him grappling with a profound emotional turmoil—a poignant example of the intricate interplay between cultural, religious, and legal factors shaping his experience.

Step 2 – Uncover

Hamid's predicament is deeply problematic within the context of Islamic teachings because, according to the Quran, his role as a husband and father carries significant responsibilities and expectations. Islamic teachings clearly outline the husband's and father's roles and emphasize their crucial obligations within the family structure.

The Quranic verse in Surah An-Nisa 4:34 underscores the husband's role as a protector and maintainer of his family: "Men are the protectors and maintainers of women." This verse signifies the husband's responsibility to safeguard and provide for his wife and children both materially and emotionally. It is his duty to ensure their well-being, which extends to being present and supportive during significant life events, such as pregnancy. Hamid's deep desire to be with Sherifa during her pregnancy aligns with the Quranic expectation of him being a protector and source of comfort for his family.

Additionally, the Quran emphasizes the importance of mutual consultation and cooperation within marriage. The Quran advises that spouses should consult each other and make decisions collectively whenever possible (Quran 42:38). This principle encourages a partnership based on mutual respect and shared responsibilities. Hamid's yearning to be with Sherifa during her pregnancy reflects his commitment to this Quranic principle, as he believes his presence is integral to fulfilling his role as a supportive husband and father.

Step 3 – Recognize

Hamid's situation presents a remarkable and atypical challenge in the realm of sex therapy. While polyamorous relationships are more commonly addressed in the field, Hamid's unique polygamous dynamic introduces distinct ethical dilemmas that demand careful consideration. Even clinicians who are generally supportive of polyamorous relationships may find themselves grappling with the concept of polygamy, raising questions about the autonomy and agency of the female partners within this multifaceted relationship. These complexities underscore the ethical intricacies that can surface when navigating non-monogamous relationships like Hamid's within the therapeutic context.

Step 4 – Develop

In formulating a therapeutic strategy to aid Hamid, it is crucial to acknowledge the boundaries inherent to the therapist's role. It is evident that the therapist has no jurisdiction or sway over government decisions regarding Hamid's second wife residing with him, or residency within the country. However, the therapist can play a pivotal role in equipping the patient with coping mechanisms for his current circumstances and potentially facilitating a reconnection with his family despite the geographical separation.

In this particular case, **psychosexual education** assumes a central role, aimed at enabling Hamid to grasp the intricacies of diverse relationship styles and emphasizing the paramount importance of effective communication within any relational context. Since Hamid and Sherifa are currently in a long-distance relationship, discussions encompassed strategies for nurturing emotional and physical intimacy, including using various communication technologies and Bluetooth-compatible sexual health aids to maintain a sense of closeness. Moreover, therapeutic sessions delved into enhancing communication skills in his relationship with Samira. Hamid's candid admission of occasional emotional shutdowns and irritability, often stemming from distress and depressive feelings, served as a foundation for addressing these challenges constructively. The focus was on equipping Hamid with tools to express his emotions effectively and manage his frustrations in a healthier and more productive manner, with the ultimate goal of fostering closeness within his relationship with Samira, rather than perpetuating division. In this instance, Samira was able to feel connected to her husband by being a source of support and encouragement to him.

Recognizing Hamid's devout Muslim background, an **integration of faith tradition** was deemed significant. In this context, several Quranic verses were found to be particularly beneficial in offering solace and guidance to Hamid, including:

Allah does not burden a soul beyond that it can bear ...
                    Surah Al-Baqarah (Quran 2:286)

Say, "Never will we be struck except by what Allah has decreed for us; He is our protector." And upon Allah let the believers rely.
                    Surah At-Tawbah (Quran 9:51)

For indeed, with hardship [will be] ease. Indeed, with hardship [will be] ease.
                    Surah Ash-Sharh (Quran 94:5–6)

And those who strive for Us – We will surely guide them to Our ways. And indeed, Allah is with the doers of good.
                    Surah Al-Ankabut (Quran 29:69)

These verses served as a wellspring of resilience and inspiration for Hamid during moments of profound emotional and spiritual depletion. They not only bolstered his resolve but also furnished him with the impetus required to persevere in his unwavering commitment to his family. While the combined approaches of psychosexual education and the integration of faith traditions yielded valuable strategies for alleviating his emotional distress, it was equally advantageous to introduce **creative solutions** tailored to those instances when he found himself grappling with exceptionally overwhelming circumstances. The following were recommended:

♦ **Emotional catharsis and self-exploration:** Hamid was actively encouraged to embrace the practice of journaling as a potent tool for the purpose of articulating and delving into his emotions, thereby unveiling any latent or unresolved feelings. This introspective exercise is intended to facilitate a deeper understanding of his emotional landscape and foster emotional healing.

♦ **Immigration assistance and family reunification:** Recognizing the complexity of his situation, Hamid was equipped with valuable resources aimed at assisting him in navigating immigration procedures. These resources are geared towards finding a viable avenue for his second wife's relocation, even in scenarios where their marital status may not hold official government recognition. This strategic step aims to mitigate the challenges stemming from familial separation.

◆ **Holistic self-care practices:** Hamid was strongly encouraged to incorporate holistic self-care routines into his daily regimen. Engaging in activities like jogging serves as an effective means to release pent-up stress and frustration, promoting not only physical well-being but also serving as an outlet for emotional catharsis. These self-care practices are integral to bolstering his overall resilience and emotional coping mechanisms.

◆ **Community engagement within his muslim network:** To further augment his spiritual well-being, it was recommended that Hamid deepen his engagement within his local Muslim community. This heightened connection can serve as a wellspring of spiritual support and guidance, enabling him to draw strength and solace from his faith tradition and the collective wisdom of his community members.

Throughout the entirety of the therapeutic journey, Hamid demonstrated remarkable engagement and wholehearted participation. His commitment to the process yielded tangible and substantial progress, evident in a notable reduction in his anxiety levels within the initial two months of therapy. A pivotal turning point emerged when, eight months after the birth of his child, Hamid's second wife successfully relocated. Remarkably, Hamid was blessed to be present in Ghana during the momentous occasion of his child's birth. In our most recent communication, Hamid conveyed a palpable sense of transformation, asserting that he now occupies a markedly improved emotional space and, crucially, has rediscovered profound meaning in his life.

Conclusion

Navigating the terrain of sex therapy with religious couples is undeniably intricate. The landscape is riddled with challenges when it comes to addressing issues related to sexual values and boundaries, particularly when individuals must reconcile their personal sexual values with those informed by their faith. The complexity deepens when non-monogamy becomes the focal point of discussion.

This chapter embarks on a profound exploration of the multi-faceted realm of non-monogamous relationship structures within the context of sex therapy, with a keen focus on the profound implications for religious patients. Offering an extensive overview encompassing various forms of non-monogamy, such as polygamy and polyamory, it undertakes an illuminating journey through three compelling case studies featuring devout individuals deeply rooted in their faith traditions—an Orthodox Jewish couple, an Apostolic Pentecostal Christian couple, and a devoted Muslim man from Ghana.

Throughout these evocative scenarios, the text underscores the formidable challenges and intricate complexities that individuals and couples grapple with as they endeavor to harmonize their faith with their intimate relationships. Whether contending with cultural norms, moral quandaries, or theological considerations, the paramount importance of a nuanced, respectful, and deeply empathetic therapeutic approach—one that seamlessly incorporates the patient's faith tradition—has been magnified. Regardless of the therapist's personal beliefs and sentiments, their mission remains resolute: to facilitate unwavering support for religious individuals as they tirelessly strive to achieve resonance between their profound spiritual convictions and the intimate dimensions of their lives. In doing so, this chapter endeavors to bridge the divide and illuminate a path toward greater understanding, empathy, and support for those traversing this complex intersection of faith, values, and intimacy within the realm of sex therapy.

References

Braida, N., Matta, E., & Paccagnella, L. (2023). Loving in consensual non-monogamies: Challenging the validity of Sternberg's triangular love scale. *Sexuality & Culture*, *27*(5), 1828–1847. DOI: 10.1007/s12119-023-10092-0

Domínguez, G. E., Pujol, J., Motzkau, J. F., & Popper, M. (2017). Suspended transitions and affective orderings: From troubled monogamy to liminal polyamory. *Theory & Psychology*, *27*(2), 183–197. DOI: 10.1177/0959354317700289

Fjeld, H. E. (2022). *The Return of Polyandry: Kinship and Marriage in Central Tibet*. Berghahn Books.

Füllgrabe, D., & Smith, D. S. (2023). "Monogamy? In this economy?": Stigma and resilience in consensual non-monogamous relationships. *Sexuality & Culture*, *27*(5), 1955–1976. DOI: 10.1007/s12119-023-10099-7

Hardy, J. W., & Easton, D. (2017). *The Ethical Slut: A Practical Guide to Polyamory, Open Relationships, and Other Freedoms in Sex and Love*, 3rd edition. Clarkson Potter/Ten Speed.

Krenawi, A. A. (2012). A study of psychological symptoms, family function, marital and life satisfactions of polygamous and monogamous women: The Palestinian case. *International Journal of Social Psychiatry*, *58*(1), 79–86. DOI: 10.1177/0020764010387063

Matsumura, K. T. (2022). Beyond polygamy. *Iowa Law Review*, *107*(5), 1903–1962.

Veaux, F., Rickert, E., & Hardy, J. W. (2014). *More Than Two: A Practical Guide to Ethical Polyamory*. Thorntree Press.

Watson, B. M., & Stein Lubrano, S. (2021). "Storming then performing": Historical non-monogamy and metamour collaboration. *Archives of Sexual Behavior*, *50*(4), 1225–1238. DOI: 10.1007/s10508-021-01926-9

12

Sexual Orientation

Introduction

For therapists specializing in the intersection of sexuality and religion, a prominent and widely discussed issue is that of sexual orientation. It can safely be assumed that this issue has become one of the most conflicting and troublesome topics in the discourse of sexuality and religion. This issue garners considerable attention in public discourse, scholarly debates, and personal disagreements. Within the realm of biblical studies, scholars often engage with the topic of sexual orientation in an attempt to either establish biblical support for or rejection of homosexuality. It is undeniable that the Hebrew Bible, the New Testament, and the Quran contain passages that could be interpreted as condemning homosexuality. However, the central question should not be whether these texts condemn homosexuality, but rather why they do so.

To gain a deeper understanding, it becomes crucial to contextualize these texts within their cultural, social, and environmental settings. Unfortunately, time and space constraints prevent us from delving into the intricacies of the exegesis process relevant to this work. This is where collaboration with biblical scholars becomes invaluable.

Nevertheless, when working with religious individuals who grapple with issues related to sexual orientation within their religious framework, a more pertinent inquiry emerges: "How do faith communities respond to them?" This question lies at the heart of the psychological, emotional, and spiritual challenges faced by those navigating

DOI: 10.4324/9781003242017-16

questions of sexual orientation or gender identity. As discussed in *Abrahamic Faiths: Perspectives on Gender Identity and Sexuality* (Jacobson, 2023), individuals seeking to understand their sexuality often find themselves in a state of inner conflict, feeling trapped and struggling to find answers that are vital for living authentically.

One of the significant factors contributing to the discord between religion and the discussion of sexual orientation, particularly, is the association between religion and conversion therapy efforts (Ogunbajo et al., 2022). It is clear that many efforts toward conversion therapy have been supported by religious institutions and movements (Ryan et al., 2020). This often makes the process of helping the patient achieve congruency between their faith and sexual orientation exceptionally difficult. This is also the area in which clinicians are most encouraged to check their bias so that it does not negatively impact the therapeutic alliance (de Oliveira Maraldi, 2020).

Therapist Bias Check

1. Is my personal understanding of sexual activity potentially diminishing the distress experienced by the patient who is struggling with an unconsummated marriage?
2. Am I applying a one-size-fits-all approach to this situation, or am I considering the unique cultural, religious, and psychological factors that may be contributing to the unconsummated marriage?

Case Study 1 – Isaac

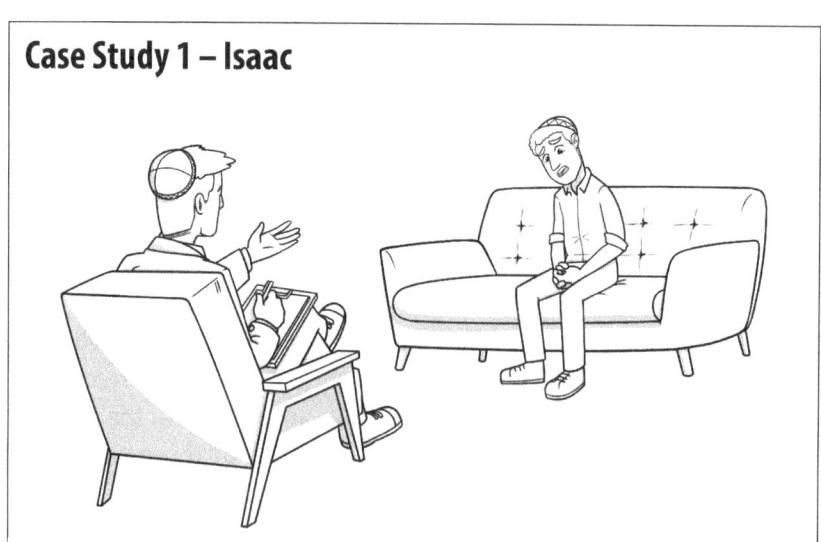

Isaac, a 20-year-old religious Orthodox Jew, is deeply entrenched in his faith. To assist him in finding a suitable life partner, his parents have engaged a matchmaker's services. During the past month, Isaac had arranged meetings with a number of potential women. The weight of these meetings has begun to manifest as intense anxiety within Isaac. His parents attribute this anxiety to his struggle to establish a genuine connection with any of the potential partners. However, Isaac confides that the source of his anxiety lies elsewhere. Starting at the young age of 12, he engaged in sexual relationships with male friends. These past experiences have instilled in him a deep-seated belief that his actions have tarnished his ability to enter into a marriage with a woman. The inner conflict between his true self and the expectations of his faith community weighs heavily on his conscience. Regarding his sexual orientation, Isaac finds himself in a state of uncertainty. The intricate interplay of emotions he navigates has left him questioning this fundamental aspect of himself.

Initial Interaction

Like many religious patients, Isaac displayed palpable anxiety during his initial session. He initially remained reticent, only responding to direct inquiries. To alleviate his concerns, I assured him of the utmost confidentiality in our sessions, emphasizing that his discussions with me would remain strictly private, undisclosed to his parents or rabbinical authorities. I proceeded to introduce the PLISSIT model, elucidating its role as our guiding framework throughout our therapeutic journey, particularly in addressing his sexual concerns. I delicately requested his permission to delve into these intimate topics, underlining that this permission-giving process was a crucial step. To further ease his nervousness, I empathetically acknowledged the difficulty of discussing such matters, especially with a new acquaintance, while emphasizing the importance of his comfort in these conversations. Isaac wholeheartedly granted permission for these discussions, and by the end of our initial session, he even expressed a sense of relief and satisfaction in being able to engage in such open dialogues.

Step 1 – Identify

Isaac was struggling to understand his sexual orientation. He had never been able to fully explore this area of himself, with the exception of early adolescent experiences. This situation was made all the more intricate due to the pervasive expectations not only from his immediate family but also from his tightly-knit religious community. These external pressures created a profound internal conflict as he attempted to reconcile his authentic self with the deeply ingrained beliefs and cultural norms that had been instilled in him from a young age.

Step 2 – Uncover

Within the specific Orthodox community of Isaac's upbringing, comprehensive sexual education was notably absent, with the exception of rigid religiously influenced sexual boundaries. Isaac was taught that masturbation was forbidden and sexual activity was only permissible when it resulted in ejaculation within the vagina. However, the onset of hormonal changes during early adolescence introduced Isaac, like all adolescents, to the stirrings of sexual desire. This led him to a period of exploration and acting upon these desires with friends of the same sex. This has been the source of internal conflict for him since those experiences.

Now, at an age where marriage becomes a prominent consideration, Isaac's family hired a matchmaker to facilitate the process, in keeping with customary practices in Orthodox communities. Nonetheless, Isaac remains burdened by intense feelings of guilt and shame stemming from his adolescent experiences. These emotions cast a shadow over his readiness to commit to a marital relationship, or if he is even worthy of marriage, adding layers of intricacy to his therapeutic journey – an intricate interplay of cultural, religious, and personal factors.

Step 3 – Recognize

Consider the multitude of ethical quandaries that can emerge in a scenario like Isaac's, each contingent on the therapist who engages with it, akin to various facets of Isaac's persona. To a non-religious therapist, the notion of restricting ejaculation exclusively to vaginal intercourse might raise concerns about

sexual freedom and autonomy. The prohibition against masturbation could appear oppressive, and the rejection of same-sex
sexual encounters might be perceived as harboring homophobic
undertones. These potential biases, while unintended, may inadvertently impact the therapeutic alliance with the patient who
holds steadfast to the values of their religious community.

In stark contrast, a religious therapist may grapple with
a sense of disappointment over Isaac's perceived inability to
adhere to his religiously informed boundaries. Their own deeply
rooted worldviews regarding sexual orientation could serve as
a barrier, hindering Isaac's exploration of his own identity in an
environment that should ideally foster freedom of self-discovery.
These divergent perspectives emphasize the intricate interplay
of ethical considerations when navigating the complex terrain of
sex therapy in a religious context.

Step 4 – Develop

As the therapeutic journey began, it was helpful to conduct a
sexual history with Isaac. This step was essential to understand
what previous experiences were causing him shame to the point
where he thought that he would never be able to get married.
During the sexual history, it was revealed that he had engaged in
sexual behavior with four guys, all of whom were around his age
at the time of the incidents. He confessed that at the time of the
encounters, he really enjoyed himself, although, after orgasm, he
often felt guilt and shame. He shared that the guys were typically his classmates, and the encounters would occur during
sleepovers or when they were alone for extended periods of
time. He estimates that these experiences stopped shortly before
his 17th birthday.

When inquired about the specific events that transpired
during these encounters, the patient revealed that they predominantly involved masturbation or mutual masturbation.
However, interspersed with these activities were occasions
where oral sex, encompassing both giving and receiving, took
place. Additionally, there were infrequent instances, numbering
two or three, where the patient underwent anal penetration,
with no corresponding engagement in such acts towards others.

Furthermore, the patient acknowledged engaging in episodes of non-ejaculatory masturbation with friends, which were not accompanied by the same level of guilt and shame that presented with the other experiences.

In the subsequent session, we shifted our focus away from discussing matters related to sexuality. In my experience, especially when working with patients who hold strong religious beliefs, delving into intricate sexual histories can often prove to be overwhelming and distressing. Therefore, the follow-up session typically adopts a less intense approach, centering on aspects related to relationships or the patient's perceptions of them.

During this session with Isaac, it came to light that he had a deep desire to build a family from a young age. Furthermore, he expressed a romantic interest in several females during his formative years and early adulthood. This information is of exceptional importance within our therapeutic process, given Isaac's profound anxiety surrounding his sexual orientation, particularly his fear of being labeled homosexual. Nevertheless, it is noteworthy that, based on his experiences, his primary attractions were directed towards females, despite his engagement in sexual interactions with males.

To encourage further introspection and exploration of Isaac's aspirations, I assigned him the task of envisioning his ideal future relationship. This assignment required him to provide a detailed description of his desired partner, covering physical attributes, personality traits, and shared interests. Additionally, Isaac was prompted to articulate the dynamics of their relationship, including the manner in which they interacted and the activities they engaged in together. Importantly, I deliberately refrained from using gender-specific language in the assignment instructions to ensure that his responses remained uninfluenced by preconceived notions.

During the subsequent session, we conducted a review of the assigned task. Isaac provided his responses to the questions presented, revealing that he had envisioned himself in a relationship with a Jewish woman possessing blonde hair and blue eyes. An interesting point emerged as he shared this information;

he disclosed that he had thought of two specific women while answering the question. Consequently, we inquired whether he held any romantic interest in these women. In response, Isaac offered a nonchalant shrug and replied, "I guess." This admission, once again, served to affirm that the underlying source of distress was considerably less related to matters of sexual orientation and far more intertwined with feelings of guilt and shame stemming from past sexual experiences.

This led the direction of therapy into **psychosexual education**. Research indicates that same-sex experiences among heterosexual individuals is not uncommon. However, in more conservative cultures, they often feel a level of discomfort, especially among heterosexual males (Nebot-Garcia et al., 2022). This, in itself, could lead to difficulties in the full development of sexuality (IsHak, 2017, 539–572). Additionally, research has long indicated that there is a high level of suicidal ideation among heterosexual adolescents with same-sex fantasies or behaviors (Zhao et al., 2010). Therefore, it could be exceptionally important to help Isaac understand the difference between sexual orientation and sexual activity. This could do two things: (1) help him better understand that his past sexual activities do not determine his sexual orientation and (2) second lesson the distress he has concerning his earlier sexual behavior.

Given Isaac's pronounced feelings of guilt stemming from his past sexual behaviors, which have created hesitations about pursuing a relationship with a potential female partner leading to marriage, it was helpful to integrate his faith tradition into our therapeutic approach in order to help him overcome these feelings of guilt and shame. In this specific case, following extensive discussions with Isaac and a thorough comprehension of the dissonance he perceives between his religious beliefs and his lived experiences, I intend to engage with him on the Jewish concepts of "sin" and "teshuvah." These discussions would have the potential to create a path toward congruency in his life.

Beginning first with the concept of "sin," I discussed with Isaac how the term is not in the Hebrew language. There are three Hebrew words that are often translated as sin, but this has primarily been for theological reasons and often the concept is interpreted from a more Christian ideal of sin than what the Hebrew text often means to imply. Take for example, the Hebrew word חטא (chet), which means to "miss the mark." This has nothing to do with eternal damnation or moral failure like the word sin so often replies. The same is true for the other two Hebrew words that are often translated as sin as well. The word עברה (avaira) means "to cross a line," and the word עון (avon) means "to bend, twist, or distort." All three of these words indicate a person's position to the religiously informed boundaries. None of these words indicate that a person is bad or evil.

With this insight, I assisted Isaac in recognizing that, even if he harbored concerns about potentially committing one of these actions, these actions do not inherently categorize him as being at enmity with God. This is where the concept of tehuvah comes in. Similar to the concept of sin, teshuvah often gets translating correctly as well. While the word is often translated as "repentance" it actually means "to return." It indicates that no matter where someone goes in their life, or what they do, they can always return. Once again, this is a term that is filled with hope, and should not be equated with fear or depravity.

Isaac derived significant emotional relief from our therapeutic conversations around faith and sexuality. They helped to facilitated a profound re-evaluation of his past behaviors. During our sessions, he shared an important revelation. While he does not experience same-sex attraction, he openly acknowledge genuine enjoyment from his past sexual experiences with individuals of the same sex during his formative years. He articulated that this enjoyment had been the primary source of his anxiety, causing him to question the feasibility of engaging in a romantic relationship with a woman.

However, as our therapeutic journey unfolded, Isaac developed a comprehensive understanding of the fluidity inherent in sexual orientation and the diverse spectrum of personal experiences. Simultaneously, he discovered solace and a deeper understanding of his faith tradition. Consequently, he experienced a newfound sense of congruency within himself. He now believes it is feasible to pursue a relationship with the potential to culminate in marriage, having harmonized his internal conflicts regarding identity and desires. Therefore, in this particular case, the **creative solution** was the use of his faith tradition to facilitate the reframing that was needed for him to feel more comfortable with himself and his previous actions thus allowing him to move forward in his life.

Following the conclusion of therapy, Isaac displayed an increased willingness to explore potential partnerships. He opted to continue therapy during the initial phase of this journey, recognizing the importance of support in navigating the adjustments and potential challenges he anticipated while embarking on the path of dating with marriage in mind. After several months of this process, he successfully connected with a partner and subsequently entered into a marital union. At the time fo this writing, the couple has been married for two and a half years and has since welcomed two children into their lives.

Case Study 2 – Michael

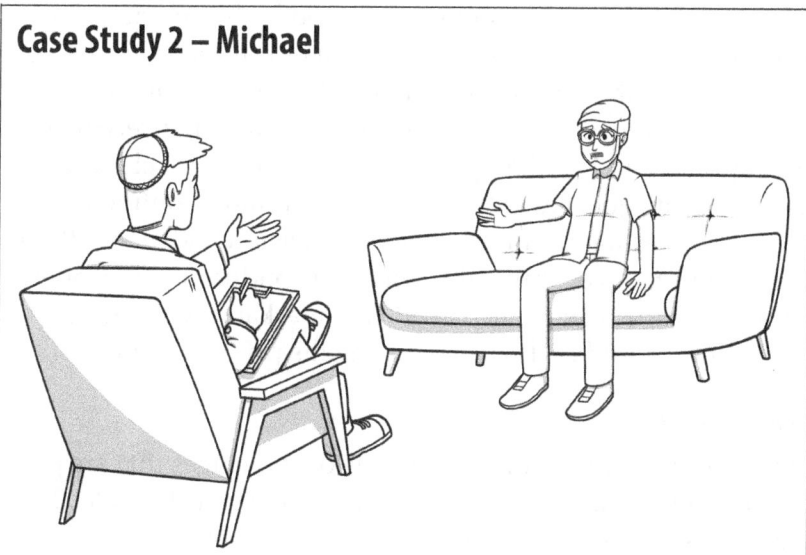

Michael is a 32-year-old man whose life revolves around his role as the music director at the Pentecostal church that his father pastors. Marrying Becky seven years ago, they've built a family with two children. However, recently, another male church member confronted Michael's father with text messages exchanged between them and Michael, revealing Michael's veiled hints at seeking sexual involvement. Michael confesses that he has been living a hidden life, engaging in various intimate encounters with men within the church and even venturing out of town to seek connections with men at adult bookstores. He has refuted the claims made by a fellow church member to his father, fearing the consequences if his same-sex desires were exposed. Losing his position as the church's music director and facing the possible dissolution of his marriage are haunting prospects that drive his fear of disclosure. Michael is struggling with his identity, faith, and desire.

Initial Interaction

When Michael initially sought therapy, he presented with a mixture of defensiveness and eagerness to engage. In our first encounter, I broached the subject of discussing sexual matters, fully cognizant of the constraints imposed by his religious background. I asked him if I could have his permission to discuss such topics with him and explained that this permission was a fundamental component of the PLISSIT model, a recognized technique within sex therapy, and underscored its relevance to his therapeutic journey. My assurance of utmost confidentiality and the suggestion for him to permit himself to delve into these sexual concerns were pivotal in setting a conducive atmosphere. Subsequently, Michael displayed a remarkable willingness to engage in a candid dialogue regarding his primary issue.

Step 1 – Identify

Michael is grappling with a multitude of challenges that are profoundly unsettling the bedrock of his well-established life. This upheaval stems from the intersection of his public and private spheres. He is contending with severe manifestations of anxiety and depression, which have cast a formidable shadow over his anticipation of the future, leaving him with a pervasive sense of losing control. Moreover, he harbors deep-seated apprehensions regarding the far-reaching implications of his recent actions on the life he has constructed, as well as on his prospects for achieving future goals.

In addition to these concerns, Michael is also confronted with a profound fear regarding the reactions of his family members. He is actively seeking strategies to mitigate potential damage to these vital relationships, reflecting his earnest desire to safeguard his familial bonds amidst the turmoil he is experiencing. Furthermore, Michael grapples with a sense of profound uncertainty surrounding his sexual orientation and habits and how these aspects may shape his future and impact his self-identity. He is in search of meaning and understanding regarding the implications of these facets of his life.

Step 2 – Uncover

Michael's situation is uniquely influenced by his conservative Christian background, which has a significant impact on his experience with his sexual orientation. As the child of a pastor and holding the position of music director within his local church, Michael occupies a prominent leadership role within his faith community. Consequently, he faces substantial expectations to uphold the established moral and ethical standards of this particular religious group. As both the minister's son and a church leader, this dual role places considerable pressure on him.

Within the framework of his religious beliefs, homosexuality is viewed as a sinful behavior, which creates internal conflict for Michael as he grapples with his sexual orientation. Adding further complexity to his situation is his marital status and the presence of children in his life. Even if he were to consider embracing a homosexual lifestyle, this would require him to get a divorce, something that his religious tradition typically does not permit. This intricate interplay of factors underscores the challenges he faces in reconciling his conservative faith with his evolving understanding of his sexual identity.

Step 3 – Recognize

Clinicians may exhibit a range of reactions to this case, influenced by their individual worldviews and belief systems, which can introduce potential bias into their therapeutic approach. Religious therapists, for example, may grapple with discomfort over Michael's involvement in same-sex relationships, particularly as he is doing so while still married to a woman, which is seen by many as an act of infidelity within certain religious contexts. This may trigger feelings of moral conflict and raise concerns about the alignment of Michael's actions with their own religious values and principles.

Conversely, non-religious therapists may be inclined to scrutinize the treatment Michael is receiving within his church community. They may harbor resentment over the implications that Michael's sexual orientation could jeopardize his role as a music leader in his father's church, viewing this as unjust and discriminatory. Additionally, they may find it disheartening and shameful that Michael potentially faces rejection from his church and family due to his sexual orientation.

These therapist biases, whether rooted in religious or non-religious perspectives, can inadvertently influence the therapeutic process and should be vigilantly recognized and managed to ensure that the treatment remains unbiased, empathetic, and aligned with the patient's best interests. It is imperative for clinicians to maintain self-awareness and actively work to mitigate any personal biases that may impede the therapeutic alliance and the patient's progress.

Step 4 – Develop

At the outset of our therapeutic collaboration, I initiated a direct discussion with Michael regarding his sexual orientation. At that time, he articulated that he believed himself to be bisexual, as he experienced romantic love for his wife. However, he disclosed that he experienced a stronger sexual attraction to individuals of the same gender, including myself. As our conversation progressed, I inquired about any past romantic involvement with other men, to which he responded negatively. This prompted further exploration into the certainty of his ability to engage in romantic relationships with other men, to which Michael expressed uncertainty.

Our dialogue then shifted towards his relationship with his wife. Michael conveyed deep affection for her, emphasizing her unwavering support, care, and exceptional role as a mother to their children. He also disclosed that their sexual activity occurred approximately once a month due to his difficulties maintaining an erection. Michael acknowledged that his wife had expressed a desire for a more active sexual life within their marriage.

During a comprehensive sexual history assessment, it came to light that Michael regularly engaged in masturbation, with infrequent use of pornography, primarily of a gay nature. He reported no issues in achieving and sustaining an erection or experiencing orgasm during solo sexual activities. Regarding past sexual experiences, Michael disclosed that his wife was the only woman he had engaged in sexual intercourse with. However, he did receive oral sex from two other females before their marriage. Notably, he revealed that since the age of 14, he had participated in a range of sexual encounters with males of varying ages. He recounted his first same-sex experience with a 19-year-old individual at a church camp, during which he engaged in oral sex and receptive penetration. He expressed enjoyment during the experience but also experienced subsequent feelings of guilt and shame.

Subsequently, I asked Michael if it was accurate to say that he derived more satisfaction from sexual encounters with men compared to his experiences with his wife, to which he affirmed.

Michael also shared that he had made several attempts to discontinue his sexual encounters with men but struggled to control his urges. He explained that this had led him to seek sexual encounters with men through various means, including dating apps, adult bookstores, and even approaching individuals within the church community and during church camp events. This revelation prompted a discussion about safer sex practices. During this conversation, I learned that he often did not use condoms in these encounters, primarily because they were typically impromptu, and he was unprepared.

At this point in our therapeutic journey, it became evident that Michael's experiences were consistent with the clinical assumption that he identified as a gay man within a heterosexual marriage. This understanding aligns with existing academic literature that highlights the importance of addressing sexual health concerns for all involved partners, particularly those who may not be aware of the situation (Ren & Yuan, 2018).

Consequently, I introduced **psychosexual education** aimed at discussing safer sex practices and the common phenomenon of gay men navigating heterosexual relationships. This served as an essential aspect of our therapeutic work.

During the initial phase of our discussions, I refrained from using the term "gay" to describe Michael. This approach aligns with my therapeutic stance that patients must self-identify, rather than accepting labels imposed upon them by a clinician. From my clinical experience, I have found that self-identification is crucial for patients to reach self-actualization. However, after approximately three months of weekly sessions, Michael eventually began referring to himself as gay. When he first used this term to describe himself, I inquired about what it meant to him. He responded by saying, "just really bad stuff." Further probing revealed that he associated his gay identity with negative outcomes. In his view, it meant he could no longer serve as the music director of his church, that he should end his marriage to his wife, and that his parents might distance themselves from him.

From Michael's responses, it became evident that his struggle was not primarily related to his personal faith but rather with his faith community. In other words, he did not express a "fear of going to hell," a sentiment commonly voiced by religious patients grappling with their gay identity. Instead, his concern revolved around how his queer identity might disrupt the social structure in which he currently lived.

At this juncture, I guided Michael toward a deeper exploration of his sexual values. I shared with him:

> *You've told me a lot about what your church thinks about sex and the values and boundaries that they have around sexual behavior, but what are yours? Do you know what your personal sexual values are? As your homework this week, I would like for you to spend time reflecting on this and write a list of what your personal sexual values are.*

In the subsequent week, Michael took the initiative to share his inventory of sexual values. Through his introspection, several recurring themes emerged, with trust and honesty being prominently featured. Seeking greater precision regarding the meaning of these terms to him, I proceeded to ask Michael whether he upheld these values consistently. His unequivocal response was "yes." However, I further probed, asking, "Even in your relationship with your wife?" This question was met with a prolonged period of silence, during which Michael began to weep. After a few moments, he raised his head and replied, "No, I haven't." This poignant moment marked a pivotal juncture in our therapeutic journey.

One day, Michael approached our therapy sessions with a strong conviction to disclose his sexual activities to his wife. Up until that point, these activities had remained the subject of rumors within their church community. Michael explained that his wife had been steadfastly defending him, even though many of the speculations were accurate. He expressed concerns about how this revelation might deeply hurt her and potentially lead to the end of their marriage. While therapy couldn't eliminate these inherent risks, it was valuable to redirect Michael's focus toward the positive aspects of his decision.

Incorporating his faith tradition into our discussion, I introduced a relevant passage from the New Testament, specifically John 15:13, which reads, "Greater love has no one than this, that someone lay down his life for his friends" (*English Standard Version*). I shared with Michael that if he genuinely loved his wife, encompassing every facet of that word, it would entail sharing important truths with her, even if these truths carried the potential for negative consequences for him. This scriptural reference served as a guiding principle to emphasize the significance of honesty and caring for his wife's well-being in this challenging situation.

Understandably, Michael was nervous and scared. He knew once he told his wife much of his behavior would become known, at least within his family. This meant that his father would find out and would most likely not allow him to continue as music minister in their church. In many of our sessions leading up to his confession to his wife, Michael was very emotional – and understandably so. There was very little that I could do or say to him that would make the situation easier or to help produce a desirable outcome. All that I could do was sit with him in his discomfort and support his decision.

During the week when Michael made the decision to have the conversation with his wife, I aimed to assist him in recognizing that even if the situation appeared challenging, he could find solace in placing his trust and faith in God. To provide support during the intervals between our sessions, I shared several relevant Scriptural references with him. I encouraged him to meditate on these Old and New Testament texts throughout the week, both leading up to his conversation with his wife and afterwards. These texts included:

Trust in the Lord with all your heart, and do not lean on your own understanding. In all your ways acknowledge him, and he will make straight your paths.
Proverbs 3:5–6 (*English Standard Version*)

Therefore I tell you, do not be anxious about your life, what you will eat or what you will drink, nor about your body, what you will put on. Is not life more than food, and the body more than clothing? Look at the birds of the air: they neither sow nor reap nor gather into barns, and yet your heavenly Father feeds them. Are you not of more value than they?
Matthew 6:25–26 (*English Standard Version*)

Come to me, all who labor and are heavy laden, and I will give you rest. Take my yoke upon you, and learn from me, for I am gentle and lowly in heart, and you will find rest for your souls. For my yoke is easy, and my burden is light.
Matthew 11:28–30 (*English Standard Version*)

Do not be anxious about anything, but in everything by prayer and supplication with thanksgiving let your requests be made known to God. And the peace of

God, which surpasses all understanding, will guard
your hearts and your minds in Christ Jesus.
Philippians 4:6–7 (*English Standard Version*)

And without faith, it is impossible to please him, for
whoever would draw near to God must believe that
he exists and that he rewards those who seek him.
Hebrews 11:6 (*English Standard Version*)

During our subsequent session, Michael displayed a profound
sense of sadness. As anticipated, his wife's reaction to the news
he had shared was far from favorable, resulting in her leaving
with their children to stay with her parents. While she had not
disclosed the reasons for her departure to her parents at that
point, Michael was aware that it was only a matter of time before
both sets of parents would become aware of the situation.

Michael expressed that if it hadn't been for the biblical texts
I had provided him and the knowledge of his upcoming therapy
appointments, he might have contemplated ending his life. This
prompted me to conduct a thorough assessment of his suicidal
tendencies. Michael assured me that he was not currently experiencing suicidal thoughts, but he acknowledged that he could
imagine such thoughts arising if he didn't have the support
network that was currently available to him. This revelation
emphasized the importance of the support structure in his life
during this challenging period.

All of Michael's initial assumptions seemed to materi-
alize into reality. Reconciliation with his wife appeared to be
an elusive prospect. The revelation of the separation reached
both his in-laws and his own parents, further compounding
the complexity of the situation. In response to this distressing
development, his father took the step of removing him from
his leadership position within the church. The resultant
embarrassment was so profound that it led Michael to discontinue attending church altogether. For several months,
the primary focus of therapy was to provide Michael with
essential support as he grappled with significant life changes

and worked through the challenges of adapting to his new circumstances.

Several months after the couple's divorce, Michael was just beginning to accept and settle into his new life as a single individual. He found spiritual support by attending another church that were more accepting of LGBTQ individuals. As per the terms of his divorce, he had his kids every other weekend and was grateful to still be a part of their life. With these major hurdles out of the way, the goal of therapy then became to help Michael develop a new relationship with his parents and navigate living as a gay male for the first time in his life.

Numerous **creative solutions** were suggested to facilitate the mending of Michael's relationship with his parents. However, their deeply rooted fundamentalist Christian beliefs posed a significant obstacle, preventing them from accepting his gay identity. They believed that their actions, marked by limited contact with him, were guided by what they perceived as "best for his soul." In their view, this approach would ultimately lead Michael back to the family fold and the religious "truth" they held dear.

Despite the challenges, I continued to encourage Michael to maintain open lines of communication with his parents whenever possible. This involved sending cards on holidays, birthdays, and anniversaries, as well as sending occasional texts and voice messages to update them on positive developments in his life. Over time, he succeeded in reestablishing a connection with his mother. However, at the time of this writing, his relationship with his father remains estranged.

At the age of 33, Michael embarked on a journey to explore and define his gay identity. He actively engaged in a wide range of community activities, including social gatherings, book clubs, and other events, with the aim of discovering where he could most authentically belong. This exploration ultimately resulted in the formation of a supportive network of friends who played a pivotal role in assisting him in the process of self-discovery, achieving self-actualization, and rekindling his zest for life.

After three and a half years of therapeutic work, Michael achieved significant milestones in his personal growth. He purchased a home, found a committed partner, and successfully launched his own photography business. These achievements underscore the transformative power of self-acceptance and the support of a nurturing community in Michael's life. Despite the fact that Michael's initial goals were unable to be achieved, he was able to find happiness, fulfillment, and finally peace of mind for the first time in his life.

Case Study 3 – Kaamil

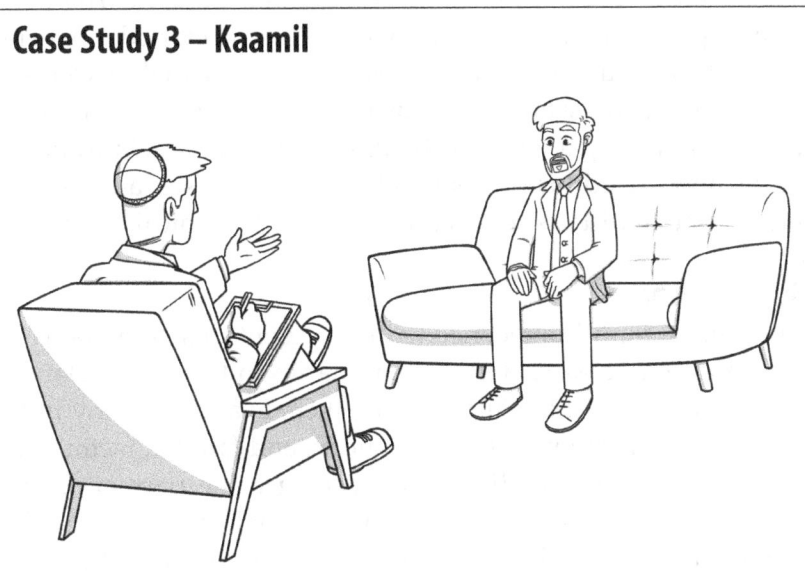

Kaamil, a 27-year-old Muslim professional working in the banking and finance sector, recently found himself facing a barrage of inquiries from his parents regarding his marital status. They've been questioning why he hasn't yet settled down with a wife. Kaamil confesses that he hasn't given much thought to his romantic life, as he's been deeply engrossed in building his career. Although he acknowledges that he's had short-lived relationships with five women in the past, none lasting longer than three or four months, he maintains that he isn't drawn to romantic involvement. While he occasionally recognizes the attractiveness of women, he doesn't feel compelled to pursue romantic connections with them. Kaamil also admits to a regular habit of masturbation, occurring three to

> four times a week. He has sought therapy primarily to address his parents' concerns, who believe something may be amiss.

Initial Interaction

Kaamil appeared very well-dressed and presented himself in a professionally poised manner during our initial session. His communication was characterized by a high degree of articulateness, suggesting that he had dedicated considerable thought to his decision to pursue therapy. It was evident that he carried a general sense of contentment and happiness in his life, with the exception of the external pressure exerted by his parents, who were insistent upon him finding a wife. As the PLISSIT model was introduced, he acknowledged his consent and gave both myself and himself permission to discuss sexual issues within the clinical setting.

Step 1 – Identify

The initial significant concern that presents itself pertains to the absence of clearly defined boundaries in Camille's relationship with his parents. Furthermore, there is a noteworthy influence stemming from cultural, religious, and familial factors that is contributing to his distress in seeking a life partner. Lastly, it is advisable to delve into Kaamil's sexual orientation, as his apparent disinterest in pursuing romantic or sexual relationships may suggest the possibility of identifying as asexual. These multifaceted issues warrant careful assessment and consideration within a clinical psychological framework.

Step 2 – Uncover

The insistence of Kaamil's parents on his pursuit of a life partner is deeply rooted in their unwavering commitment to religious doctrines that underscore the centrality of marriage as an integral source of happiness and life fulfillment. Their devout adherence to Islam propels them to perceive it as not only their obligation but also a moral imperative to actively assist their son in finding a prospective spouse, aligning with the precepts of their faith. This complex issue primarily revolves around the intricate interplay of his religious beliefs, personal identity, and familial expectations.

It is imperative to acknowledge that Kaamil's potential sexual orientation may be perceived as divergent from the traditional gender roles prescribed for Muslim men. This divergence may introduce intricate and nuanced challenges, as well as complexities associated with cultural and religious anticipations that have the potential to profoundly affect his self-identity and overall experience. Furthermore, it could precipitate familial discord, as his parents may encounter difficulties in comprehending and accepting his choices concerning matters related to sexuality and matrimony.

Step 3 – Recognize

Clinicians may encounter various forms of bias when working with individuals of diverse religious backgrounds and sexual orientations. Such biases can emanate from both religious and nonreligious beliefs and perspectives on sexual orientation. Therapists, irrespective of their own religious affiliation, might encounter challenges in comprehending and accepting certain sexual orientations as integral components of the broader spectrum. Religious therapists may find it challenging to understand deviations from traditional gender roles, which are often prominent within conservative religious communities. On the other hand, non-religious therapists might struggle with the dynamics involving the patient's parents, as they may perceive the parents as exerting undue influence by imposing religious values and ideals upon their child. These biases and complexities warrant careful consideration and a culturally informed approach within the clinical context.

Step 4 – Develop

In the initial phases of therapy, Kaamil grappled with profound confusion and uncertainty. He found himself perplexed by the stark contrast between his remarkable success in the business realm and his perceived failure in establishing meaningful relationships. This discrepancy was compounded by his sense of non-prioritization of romantic connections, which diverged from societal and religious expectations and the experiences of his peers and family. The repeated words of concern from his parents and friends further reinforced the notion that something might be psychologically amiss, a belief he internalized and which ultimately drove him to seek therapeutic assistance.

At the beginning of the therapeutic approach, the primary focus was on gaining insights into Kaamil's sexuality. While his discussions during the assessment phase suggested the possibility of him identifying as asexual, it became evident that he was unfamiliar with this term. Therefore, it became apparent early on that **psychosexual education** was a critical component of our work, as Kaamil possessed limited knowledge regarding various relationship styles and dynamics. His understanding of sexual orientation was largely confined to the binary concepts of "gay" or "straight." This limitation was not surprising, given that these topics are typically absent from educational and religious contexts, the two primary spheres where Kaamil would have encountered such information (Rothblum et al., 2019).

Through our ongoing conversations and his shared experiences, it appeared increasingly likely that Kaamil identified as asexual. Moreover, the emotional and psychological distress that led him to seek therapy closely mirrored the experiences of asexual individuals, as corroborated by existing literature (Chan & Leung, 2023). However, I maintained a cautious approach, refraining from imposing any labels or identities onto Kaamil, as it was essential for him to arrive at these conclusions autonomously. In working with patients exploring their sexual orientations, my goal has always been to facilitate their self-discovery by helping them articulate their sexual interests, values, and boundaries, irrespective of external familial or religious frameworks, ultimately helping the patient reach self-actualization.

In this specific case, I deemed it beneficial to incorporate Kaamil's religious tradition as an initial step toward our shared objective. I assigned him reflective homework that required him to elucidate what his Islamic faith taught about his individual identity. In essence, this task prompted him to contemplate the Quranic teachings and the wisdom of the Prophet concerning the essence of a person, their relationship with Allah, and the purpose of life. This exercise laid the groundwork for pivotal concepts that would subsequently frame our therapeutic journey.

To the question of: *When did man's relationship to Allah begin?* Kaamil introduced the following passage:

O People, if you should be in doubt about the Resurrection, then [consider that] indeed, We created you from dust, then from a sperm-drop, then from a clinging clot, and then from a lump of flesh, formed and unformed – that We may show you. And We settle in the wombs whom We will for a specified term, then We bring you out as a child, and then [We develop you] that you may reach your [time of] maturity. And among you is he who is taken in [early] death, and among you is he who is returned to the most decrepit [old] age so that he knows, after [once having] knowledge, nothing. And you see the earth barren, but when We send down upon it rain, it quivers and swells and grows [something] of every beautiful kind.

Surah Al-Hajj (Quran 22:5)

This verse highlighted the Islamic teaching that Allah was a part of the entire creation and birth process. This can be understood that Kaamil was created by Allah. This is when I posed the question, *Does Allah Make Mistakes?* To which he stated, "no." He also shared passages emphasizing that Allah knows everything, such as Surah Al-Hadid (Quran 57:4) and Surah Al-Baqarah (Quran 2:225). The discussion was then moved to *According to Islam, why are we born?* To this, the following ayah were shared:

◆ *To worship Allah.*

And I did not create the jinn and mankind except to worship Me.

Surah Adh-Dhariyat (Quran 51:56)

This verse suggests that the ultimate purpose of human existence is to worship and serve Allah.

◆ *To be stewards of the earth.*

And [mention, O Muhammad], when your Lord said to the angels, "I will create a vicegerent on earth." They said, "Will You place upon it one who causes corruption therein and sheds blood, while we declare Your praise and sanctify You?" Allah said, "Indeed, I know that which you do not know."

Surah Al-Baqarah (Quran 2:30)

This ayah indicates that humans are created as vicegerents or stewards on Earth and are responsible for maintaining the balance and order on the planet.

◆ *To seek knowledge and understanding.*

 Allah will exalt in degree those of you who believe and those who have been granted knowledge.

Surah Al-Mujadila (Quran 58:11)

This ayah recognizes the value of both faith and knowledge and suggests that those with knowledge are elevated in status.

These Quranic passages served as a foundational framework for the work with Kaamil. They underscore the significance of knowledge and understanding within the Islamic context, suggesting that seeking knowledge and understanding about oneself is not only encouraged but considered a paramount endeavor. This concept would be used to motivate and challenge Kaamil in our therapeutic work.

Additionally, the Quranic belief that Allah created mankind individually and without error is a crucial point of reference. It serves as a counterpoint to Kaamil's self-perceived flaws and doubts about himself. By recognizing that Allah's creation is perfect and without fault, Kaamil can challenge the assumption that there is something inherently wrong or flawed about his own being. Thus, by using these passages it is possible to **incorporate his faith tradition** to promote self-acceptance, self-understanding, and the pursuit of personal growth and knowledge within the context of Kaamil's Islamic faith.

The next step was to help Kaamil understand his sexual values, beliefs, and ideals. I explained the homework in the following way:

♦ *I want to know what your sexual values are. Everyone says they have values, but few people ever stop to think what they are. So, I want you to make a list about what your personal values around sex are. Don't tell me what Islam says, or what your family says, I want to know what you personally think.*

In the subsequent session, Kaamil articulated his sexual values, highlighting his significant emphasis on the nuclear family structure. He defined this as comprising a union between a man and a woman, with the primary purpose of producing offspring. When queried about whether sexual activity should be confined solely to the context of marriage, he expressed a nuanced viewpoint, indicating that it is not an absolute requirement. He elaborated that if two individuals genuinely love and care for each other, he considers it acceptable for them to engage in sexual relations outside of marriage.

However, it's noteworthy that while Kaamil outlined these values regarding sexual relationships, he concurrently conveyed a relatively low level of personal interest in sexual activities and a lack of enthusiasm for the prospect of marriage. This intricate interplay of values and personal preferences provides valuable insights into Kaamil's outlook on relationships and intimacy, which warrant further exploration in our therapeutic journey.

Consequently, I engaged Kaamil in a direct and candid manner, posing a straightforward question regarding his sexual orientation by asking if he identified as gay. Following a brief pause of contemplation, he responded definitively, stating that he was not gay. This exchange represented a pivotal moment in our discussions, shedding light on an important aspect of Kaamil's self-perception and identity. Therefore, I asked him, "So, how do you identify sexually?"

As a result of the prior psychosexual education, Kaamil had acquired a more comprehensive understanding of the spectrum of sexual orientations, which empowered him to challenge his previously held beliefs and concepts. Within the therapeutic setting, he felt secure and open to exploring these aspects of his identity. During our discussions, Kaamil initially identified as heterosexual, but he began to realize that he lacked significant sexual or romantic interest in women. Subsequently, he posed the question of whether he might be asexual.

In response to his inquiry, I explained that determining his sexual orientation was a personal journey that only he could undertake. I encouraged him to reflect on what it would mean for him if he were asexual and how it might impact his life. Kaamil initially expressed uncertainty about the implications, but after thoughtful consideration, he recognized that adopting an asexual identity would resonate with his current feelings and experiences. Importantly, he acknowledged that it would alleviate the pressure he felt to conform to his parents' expectations for his future.

Over the course of three weeks, Kaamil and I delved deeply into the exploration of his asexuality and the significance of embracing this identity. The process of asexual identity development involves self-questioning, and therefore I wanted to challenge Kaamil to question his held heterosexual perspectives and have more awareness of his desires, behaviors, and attractions (Kelleher & Murphy, 2022). In a particularly poignant and emotionally charged session, Kaamil tearfully declared that he identified as asexual. This revelation, marked by a rare display of vulnerability, marked a pivotal moment in his therapeutic journey. It granted him a profound sense of self-understanding and acceptance, facilitating his emotional growth and well-being.

The concluding phase of asexual identity development includes personal identity acceptance and disclosure to others (Kelleher & Murphy, 2022). For Kaamil, the aspect of disclosure was exceptionally important since much of the distress that he was facing was coming from the pressure his family was putting on him to get married. Therefore, as part of strategizing how to effectively communicate this newfound aspect of Kaamil's identity to his parents, **creative suggestions** were given to help him have an open discussion with them. It was imperative that this communication be conducted in a manner that would facilitate their understanding and reduce the pressure they were exerting on him to enter into a traditional marriage.

While open, honest, and heartfelt communication was emphasized, a few other suggestions were given:

♦ **Seek guidance from religious leaders:** I advised Kaamil to consider reaching out to a respected religious leader within his community for guidance and support. I explained that this religious leader could offer valuable insights and help Kaamil navigate the conversation about his asexuality with his parents, given their shared faith.

♦ **Communicate with empathy:** I stressed the significance of approaching the conversation with empathy and understanding. I explained to Kaamil that he should acknowledge that this may be a challenging topic for his parents to accept and convey his genuine appreciation for their feelings and perspectives.

♦ **Framing within faith:** I encouraged Kaamil to articulate how his asexuality is aligned with his faith and deeply held values. I explained that he could emphasize that Islam promotes self-awareness and authenticity, illustrating how he is striving to live in accordance with these fundamental principles.

♦ **Highlight shared values:** I suggested to Kaamil the importance of highlighting the values he shares with his parents, including their faith, commitment to family, and love. I explained that he could reassure them that his asexuality does not diminish his dedication to these cherished values, thereby providing them with comfort and understanding.

♦ **Gradual disclosure:** I recommended to Kaamil the idea of a gradual disclosure approach, especially if he believed that his parents might initially struggle with the concept. I explained that he could begin by discussing his asexuality and then gradually introduce the topic of marriage over a series of conversations, allowing his parents time to process and adjust to this significant aspect of his identity.

Ultimately, Kaamil successfully engaged in a heartfelt and candid conversation with his parents, disclosing his asexual identity. During this conversation, his parents posed numerous questions and conveyed their concerns regarding the implications of his identity for his future. Predominantly, they expressed apprehension about the possibility that Kaamil might later change his mind, making it challenging for him to pursue a traditional marriage. They also voiced concerns about his potential loneliness in later years. However, Kaamil revealed that the most challenging aspect for his parents to accept was the realization that they might not have grandchildren from him. Notwithstanding these concerns, Kaamil conveyed that his family expressed unwavering love for him and a steadfast commitment to supporting him, irrespective of the choices he made regarding his personal life.

In our concluding session, Kaamil conveyed profound gratitude for the therapeutic journey we embarked upon. He expressed a newfound sense of comfort and self-assuredness in his adult identity, marking a significant transformation in his life. This attainment of self-actualization not only bolstered his confidence but also had a positive ripple effect on various other facets of his life, notably his professional endeavors. Nevertheless, what held the most profound significance for Kaamil was the realization and acknowledgment of the profound love and unwavering commitment his family held for him. Throughout this therapeutic process, the bonds of connection with his family were not only preserved but deepened, a deeply cherished outcome for him.

Conclusion

Navigating the intersection of sexual orientation and conservative faith presents a challenging terrain for sex therapists. Notably, fundamentalist sects within the Christian church have taken a firm stance against anything diverging from heterosexual relationships, resulting in profound identity struggles for many individuals within these communities. This issue often appears to create a seemingly irreconcilable tension between one's faith and one's sexual orientation.

It is not uncommon for individuals from all three Abrahamic faith traditions to seek therapy for concerns related to their sexual orientation. Paradoxically, this is an area where many sex therapists may encounter difficulties when working with religious patients. The challenges may stem from the association between conversion therapy and certain religious communities (Ogunbajo et al., 2022), and the well-documented adverse outcomes associated with conversion therapy, including depression, suicidal thoughts, suicide attempts, lower educational attainment, and reduced income (Ryan et al., 2020). However, it remains the ethical duty of mental health professionals to approach these individuals with compassion and empathy while respecting their autonomy over their beliefs and sexual behavior.

The three case studies presented in this chapter serve to underscore the critical importance of integrating an individual's deeply held religious beliefs into the therapeutic process when addressing issues related to sexual orientation. Whether the patient chooses to depart from their faith community or embraces practices that may raise concerns from a professional standpoint, it is imperative that we acknowledge and respect their rights as autonomous individuals. This includes the right to make choices that align with their personal convictions, while also recognizing the potential complexities and internal conflicts they may grapple with in the process of reconciling their faith and sexual identity.

References

Chan, R. C.H., & Leung, J. S.Y. (2023). Experiences of minority stress and their impact on suicidality among asexual individuals. *Journal of Affective Disorders, 325,* 794–803. DOI: 10.1016/j.jad.2023.01.025

de Oliveira Maraldi, E. (2020). Response bias in research on religion, spirituality and mental health: A critical review of the literature and methodological recommendations. *Journal of Religion and Health, 59*(2), 772–783. DOI: 10.1007/s10943-018-0639-6

IsHak, W. W. (Ed.). (2017). *The Textbook of Clinical Sexual Medicine*. Springer International Publishing.

Jacobson, C. (2023). *Abrahamic Faiths: Perspectives on Gender Identity and Sexuality*, 2nd edition. Scholars' Press.

Kelleher, S., & Murphy, M. (2022). Asexual identity development and internalisation: A thematic analysis. *Sexual and Relationship Therapy*, 1–29. DOI: 10.1080/14681994.2022.2091127

Nebot-Garcia, J. E., Giménez-García, C., García-Barba, M., Gil-Llario, M. D., & Ballester-Arnal, R. (2022). What does heterosexuality mean? same-sex attraction, behaviors, and discomfort among self-identified heterosexual young adults from Spain. *Archives of Sexual Behavior*, *51*(7), 3431–3442. DOI: 10.1007/s10508-022-02315-6

Ogunbajo, A., Oke, T., Abubakari, G. M., & Oginni, O. (2022). Religiosity and conversion therapy is associated with psychosocial health problems among sexual minority men (SMM) in Nigeria. *Journal of Religion and Health*, *61*(4), 3098–3128. DOI: 10.1007/s10943-021-01400-9

Ren, Z., & Yuan, C. (2018). Mental health professionals' ethical dilemma when working with gay men who are in heterosexual marriages in China. *Journal of Gay & Lesbian Mental Health*, *22*(3), 302–307. DOI: 10.1080/19359705.2018.1463884

Rothblum, E. D., Heimann, K., & Carpenter, K. (2019). The lives of asexual individuals outside of sexual and romantic relationships: Education, occupation, religion and community. *Psychology and Sexuality*, *10*(1), 83–93. DOI: 10.1080/19419899.2018.1552186

Ryan, C., Toomey, R. B., Diaz, R. M., & Russell, S. T. (2020). Parent-initiated sexual orientation change efforts with LGBT adolescents: Implications for young adult mental health and adjustment. *Journal of Homosexuality*, *67*(2), 159–173. DOI: 10.1080/00918369.2018.1538407

Zhao, Y., Montoro, R., Igartua, K., & Thombs, B. D. (2010). Suicidal ideation and attempt among adolescents reporting "Unsure" sexual identity or heterosexual identity plus same-sex attraction or behavior: Forgotten groups? *Journal of the American Academy of Child and Adolescent Psychiatry*, *49*(2), 104–113. DOI: 10.1016/j.jaac.2009.11.003

PART IV

From Personal Bias to Professional Growth

Overview

Acknowledging personal biases presents a crucial avenue for personal and professional development. This section meticulously delineates numerous domains for such growth, offering practical guidance on their integration. Furthermore, clinicians are impassioned to persist in their work with religious patients, embracing this journey of growth as an inherent aspect of their professional evolution.

Learning Objectives

◆ Acknowledge areas of personal bias toward religion/religious individuals.
◆ Explore ways that bias can lead to personal and professional development.
◆ Question the possibility of personal spiritual growth.
◆ Develop multiple worldviews.

DOI: 10.4324/9781003242017-17

13

The Problem with Religious Patients

Introduction

While it may be perceived as exceptionally blunt, the problem with religious patients is that they probably hold views and beliefs that are the polar opposite of our own. This reality can manifest itself very quickly and hit us very forcefully. Sometimes, this can come as a complete surprise while other times, the clinician nervously waits, dreading the moment when something triggering is said or done. It is in these moments that a clinician's bias can begin to enter into the therapeutic setting and create problematic outcomes for not only the therapeutic alliance as a whole but both the patient and the clinician individually.

In Chapter 1 of this book, I discussed the three ways therapist bias manifests itself in the clinical setting. Specifically, it looked at how bias manifests itself when a non-religious clinician works with a religious patient. Nevertheless, this is not the only scenario that may transpire. Bias can also manifest itself when a religious therapist sees a religious patient, regardless if they share the same or different faith traditions. Not to mention the bias that can occur when a religious clinician works with a non-religious patient. The conflict can, of course, go both ways as the patient can have their own biases against the clinician based upon their

DOI: 10.4324/9781003242017-18

religion or based on their lack of religious ideologies. This is the case whenever there is a clash of multi-complex identities.

As a helping professional, it is necessary to take into account biases and the impact that they have on the therapeutic alliance. By better understanding the dynamics in which bias can manifest, the clinician can recognize its presence early, making it possible to resolve such conflicts before they consciously interfere with the clinician-patient relationship. The process of identifying potential biases is known as **bias awareness**, and the process of working through potential conflicts is known as **bias resolution**.

Bias Awareness

Due to the complex nature and diversity within religious communities, as well as within various faith traditions, it would be exceptionally difficult to create a stand-alone inventory to measure clinician bias when working with religious patients. Nevertheless, we can and should aim for bias awareness. Bias awareness is when the clinician has taken the time to reflect on possible problematic topics, issues, and situations that could arise when working with a specific population.

Religion and spirituality can enter the therapeutic process in multiple ways (Duggal & Sriram, 2022). Therefore, the clinician must be aware of not only their bias but also the possibility of the patient's bias and how it could manifest in the therapeutic relationship depending on the identities of all parties involved. Often, therapists are informed of the possibility of their own biases and perhaps have discovered ways to deal with their biases. Yet they often do not consider the possibility of patient's bias, nor consider ways of addressing it. There are three possible scenarios for either form of bias to manifest: (1) non-religious therapist/religious patient, (2) religious therapist/religious patient, and (3) religious therapist/non-religious patient. All three of these relationships feature unique dynamics for multi-directional bias manifestation. It is only with awareness that such dynamics exist that one can proactively aim to reduce the possibility of problematic attitudes, beliefs, and behaviors from hindering the clinician-patient relationship.

Non-Religious Therapist/Religious Patient

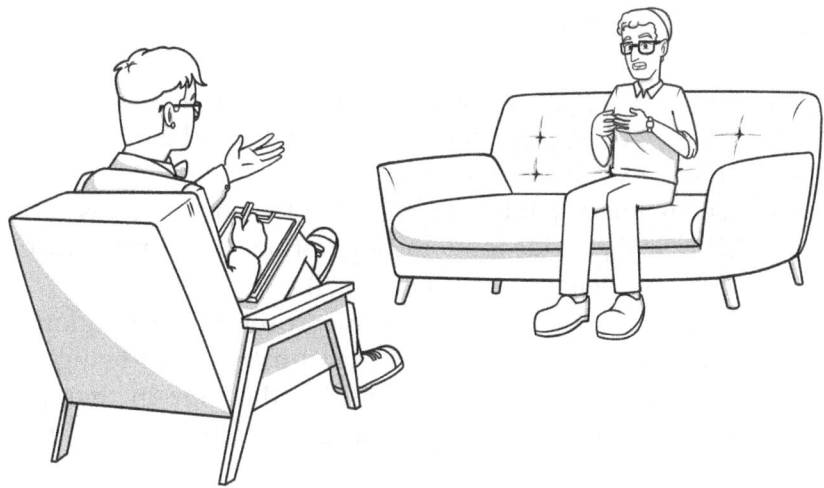

Perhaps for any people reading this book, the central conflicting relationship that comes to mind is that of a non-religious therapist working with a religious patient. During the course of their interactions, the religious patient will no doubt say things that could be triggering to the non-religious therapist. These remarks could be triggering in multiple ways:

◆ The therapist, who is now non-religious, may have experienced some form of religious trauma in the past. Hearing the patient talk about their personal experience related to sexuality and religion becomes retraumatizing for the clinician.

◆ If the therapist holds more permissive views on topics related to sexual expression, sexual identity, and sexual orientation, for example, than those of the patient, the patient's religiously informed beliefs on these topics can be triggering.

◆ If the non-religious therapist has negative opinions about religion or a specific religious tradition, microaggressions can manifest when the patient talks about spiritual things.

Likewise, there could be bias on the part of the religious patient when working with a non-religious fight therapist. This can also appear in several forms:

♦ The religious patient believes that the clinician will be dismissive of their religion or ridicule their religious beliefs (Grey et al., 2020).
♦ The religious patient believes that the non-religious clinician will provide immoral suggestions that counter their religious beliefs (Grey et al., 2020).
♦ Some religious patients from proselytizing religions, may be concerned about the spiritual well-being of the clinician, and seek to utilize the time in therapy to affect change and spiritual growth in the life of the therapist.

Religious Therapist/Religious Patient

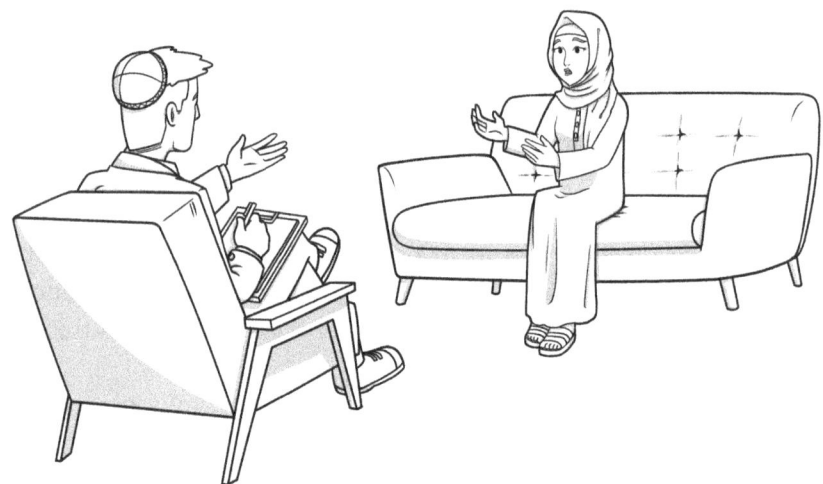

While it may seem that the best scenario would be to have a religious therapist and a religious patient, this is not always the case. Disclosure of the therapist's religious status has the potential to either strengthen the therapeutic alliance or cause discomfort (Magaldi & Trub, 2018). For example, studies show that conservative Christians prefer working with Christian therapists

(Salem & Hijazi, 2019). However, other studies show that Muslim patients sometimes prefer working with therapists who are not Muslim (Grey et al., 2020).

Spero (1985) was among the first to discuss the common countertransferential and transferential issues that could arise when religious clinicians work with religious patients. Abernethy and Lancia (1998) offered four types of transference and countertransference:

> **Interreligious transference** may emerge when the patient perceives that the therapist and the patient have different religious backgrounds. **Intrareligious transference** may occur when the patient perceives that the therapist and patient have similar religious backgrounds. **Interreligious countertransference** may happen when the therapist perceives that the therapist and patient have different religious backgrounds. **Intrareligious countertransference** may emerge when the therapist perceives that the therapist and patient have similar religious backgrounds.

In these instances, bias on the part of the clinician may appear in the following ways:

◆ During interreligious countertransference, the clinician may feel that the patient has incorrect or faulty religious beliefs and may feel the need to correct the patient's belief system. While this occurs when the clinician and patient come from two completely different faith traditions, it is also ubiquitous when they are members of other sects of the same faith tradition.

◆ During intrareligious countertransference, the clinician may judge the patient based on their behavior or thoughts, assuming that because of their faith tradition, they should "know better."

Similarly, bias on the patient may appear as follows:

◆ During interreligious transference, the patient may feel as though the clinician is judging them for being of an alternative faith tradition. Or, is either offering suggestions that are counter to the patient's religious tradition or offering suggestions that promote the clinician's religious belief system.

♦ During intrareligious transference, the patient may feel as though the clinician is judging them for not living up to the standard of their faith tradition. Or, they may fear that sensitive information is compromised and others within their faith community will find out if the clinician were to tell someone or possibly inform the clergy.

Religious Therapist/Non-Religious Patient

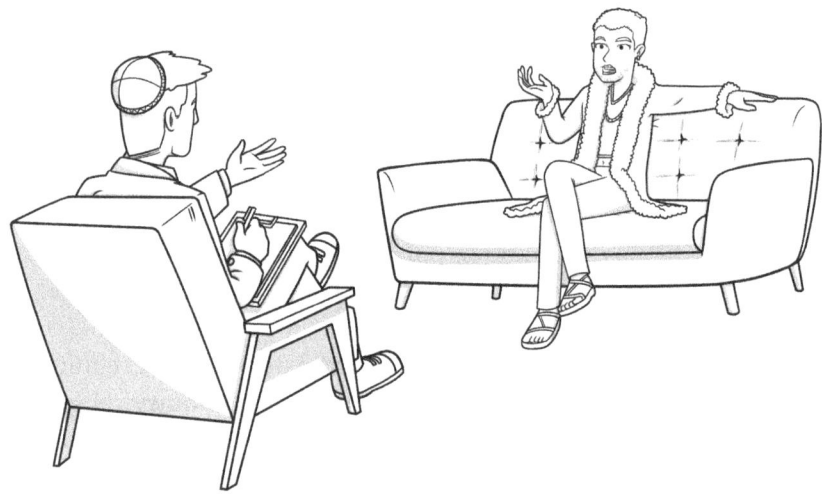

While a therapist must remain as neutral as possible, their religion does inform the way that they practice (Duggal & Sriram, 2022). As an Orthodox Jew, for example, I have often said in interviews that my religious belief system has shaped my therapeutic outlook. The example I often give is the Jewish principle of **Tikkun Olam**, the concept of repairing the world, as the motivation for my work. This motivation demonstrates the positive impact religion has on clinical practice. However, while religion can positively impact a clinician's practice, the clinician's faith could also impact their bias.

A religious therapist can have a bias against non-religious patients in the following ways:

◆ The religious therapist could feel sorry or pity their non-religious patient due to what they perceive as a lack of spiritual development.
◆ The religious therapist could project their religiously informed morals on the non-religious patient.
◆ The religious therapist could be judgmental or disappointed in the non-religious patient if they discover that the patient once belonged to the same religious tradition.

The non-religious patient can also have a bias against the therapist if they discover that the therapist is religious. This can take place for numerous reasons:

◆ The non-religious patient has negative views and ideas concerning religion, which are projected upon the therapist.
◆ The non-religious patient feels the therapist is projecting morals upon them or offering unwanted religious intervention (Byrne et al., 2021).
◆ The non-religious patient feels that the religious clinician judges them based on their lack of religious observance.

Bias Resolution

When working with religious patients, therapists need to be aware of the possibility of bias. Bias can manifest differently, such as through stereotyping or assumptions based on the patient's religion. This bias can affect the therapeutic relationship and hinder the patient's progress. However, by taking specific steps, therapists can reduce the severity of the bias and improve the quality of care they provide to their patients.

The process of reducing bias is known as bias resolution. It involves identifying and addressing any biased attitudes or beliefs that may exist on the part of the therapist or the patient. One way to achieve bias resolution is through self-reflection. Therapists can examine their own biases and beliefs, and consider how these may influence their interactions with patients. By acknowledging their biases, therapists can take the necessary steps to avoid making assumptions or judgments about their patients based on their religion.

Another strategy for bias resolution is to engage in cultural competence training. This involves learning about the different cultures and religions that patients may belong to and developing an understanding of their beliefs and practices. By doing so, therapists can provide more effective treatment that is tailored to the specific needs and values of each patient.

Finally, therapists can work collaboratively with their patients to address any potential biases. This can involve encouraging open and honest communication about any concerns or misunderstandings related to religion. By creating a safe and non-judgmental environment, therapists can help patients feel more comfortable discussing sensitive topics related to their faith.

Overall, bias resolution is an important aspect of providing effective therapy to religious patients. By being aware of and addressing biases that may arise, therapists can build stronger relationships with their patients and provide more effective treatment that respects their religious beliefs and practices.

Suggestions for Resolving Therapist's Bias

For therapists who discover that they have a bias toward their religious patient, it is crucial for them first to identify the underlying cause of such bias. Only after pinpointing the source of the bias can they take appropriate measures to address it. Once identified, the clinician can utilize the following suggestions:

♦ **Religious education.** Taking courses or reading books written from the perspective of the patient's religious tradition can be helpful in understanding the faith tradition in a way that is not pathologizing or critical. You can also get further insight into the patient's religious tradition, which can be helpful in better understanding the patient and implementing aspects of their religious beliefs into the therapeutic process.

♦ **Develop religious appreciation.** Similar to developing cultural appreciation, one can establish religious appreciation by watching films, attending religious events, such as services, and celebrating religious holidays. Doing this can also help the clinician relate more to the patient through shared experiences.

♦ **Seek training.** A clinician may wish to take specialized training and work with religious individuals or professional trainings that highlights the disparity and marginalization of many religious communities. Such courses can introduce the clinician to current research that could be helpful in their practice, as well as provide an opportunity for them to learn and grow with instructors and fellow learners.

♦ **Supervision.** One way to ensure that bias does not impact the therapeutic relationship is supervision. Within clinical supervision, the therapist can discuss with their supervisor the struggles they are having working with the religious patient and the negative feelings and emotions being brought up. Collectively, the therapist and supervisor can work together to resolve the clinician's bias.

♦ **Consultation.** The therapist may also wish to seek consultation with religious leaders or religious scholars. This will be an appropriate time for the therapist to ask very direct and possibly negative leaning questions. Due to the experience and training of the scholars and religious leaders, they would be more prepared and equipped to answer such questions than the patient, who would typically have much less knowledge and understanding of apologetics and theology.

Suggestions for Resolving Patient's Bias

When a patient's bias affects the therapeutic relationship, resolving it can be challenging for the clinician. However, there are still some options to consider.

One approach is to address the bias directly with the patient. Although it may seem confrontational, the clinician can empower the therapeutic process by asking the patient about their perceived bias. It's important to use tact when bringing up the subject. For example, the clinician might say, "I've noticed you seem a little distant or hostile during our discussion. Can you tell me more about what you're dealing with internally?"

Another option is to consult with a clergy member of the patient's faith tradition. However, it's important to note that the clinician should not seek out the patient's own clergy without their consent, as this could be seen as an act of betrayal and disrupt the development of trust. Instead, consulting with a clergyperson of the same faith tradition can help the clinician gain skills to more appropriately address the patient's concerns from a religious perspective. This could lead to a deeper understanding of the patient's worldview and facilitate more effective communication.

Addressing a patient's bias can be a difficult task for clinicians. However, by directly addressing the issue with the patient and consulting with a clergy member of the same faith tradition, clinicians can gain a better understanding of the patient's perspective and develop strategies for addressing their concerns. These approaches may help to build trust and promote a more effective therapeutic relationship.

Of course, in a perfect world, no bias would exist in any of our therapeutic relationships. However, the reality is that bias is often present, regardless of whether we choose to acknowledge it or not. As helping professionals, we have a choice: we can recognize our bias and put forth the effort to resolve it, we can ignore our bias and hinder our professional development, or we can transfer our bias and assert that the patient is at fault. While these are all possible options when bias manifests in therapy, there are things that can be done to limit the likelihood of conflict between therapist and patient.

One such approach is to engage in ongoing self-reflection and examination of our own biases, assumptions, and values. This can help us become more aware of our blind spots and work to mitigate them in our therapeutic work. Additionally, building a solid therapeutic alliance based on trust, empathy, and active listening can help to create a safe and open space for patients to share their experiences and perspectives, even when they differ from our own. Finally, seeking continuing education and training in cultural competence and diversity can help us become more effective and informed clinicians, able to navigate the complexities of bias and diversity in therapy. By taking these steps, we can work towards creating a more inclusive, understanding, and effective therapeutic environment for all patients.

What to Avoid When Working with Religious Patients

Due to the multi-directional bias projections that religion introduces into the therapeutic relationship, it is of the utmost importance that the therapist is mindful of the approaches and techniques that are employed within each session. It is equally as important to be mindful of what you don't do as it is what you will do. There are several things that should be avoided when working with religious patients. By avoiding these pitfalls, the clinician can help reduce the bias on the patient's part and reduce the perceived bias projected upon the patient.

Assumptions
It should go without saying that therapists should avoid assumptions when working with any population. However, it is sometimes very easy to get into the habit of assuming things about those who adhere to religious practices. Sometimes, these assumptions are not made with ill intent. Due simply to the magnitude of diversity within various faith traditions, as well as personal levels of observance, assumptions related to a person's religious beliefs, and the impact of those beliefs.

Microaggressions
Microaggressions are "derogatory slights or insults directed at a target person or persons who are members of an oppressed group" (Sue et al., 2019, 3). While this definition uses the phrase "oppressed group," I suggest that microaggressions are better understood as derogatory slights or insults directed at a target

person or persons who are members of a marginalized group. This would also include religious communities and faith traditions. In fact, recent research has identified religious microaggressions as a common problem in psychotherapy (Trusty et al., 2022). Microaggressions can be delivered both implicitly and explicitly, and in either case, bias is communicated (Sue et al., 2019, 3). Therefore, sex therapists should be extra careful to avoid any religious microaggressions.

Theological Arguments

Getting involved in a theological discussion with a patient who has not been theologically trained in biblical languages, as a therapist who has not been trained in biblical languages, against a pastor who most likely has not been trained in biblical languages is a disaster and should be avoided at all costs. The result is just confusion, frustration, and crisis on the part of the patient. It also introduces conflict within the therapeutic alignment that may be impossible to overcome. When forced to choose between believing their clergy, whom they have known for a long time, or a clinician that they have known for a short time or possibly just met, the clinician will lose out each time. This is a senseless and pointless exercise that only demonstrates the clinician's bias and hubris.

The Importance of Clinician Boundaries

In Chapter 2, we emphasized the importance of respecting religious patients' boundaries regarding sex, sexuality, and gender. However, as clinicians, we also need to recognize and respect our own boundaries to avoid ethical dilemmas and ensure that our personal biases don't affect the therapy session.

It's perfectly acceptable to have different opinions from our patients, just as we don't need to impose our views on them. We can appreciate and respect their worldview and beliefs without adopting them as our own. Clinicians and patients can have different perspectives and still achieve positive therapeutic outcomes. As clinicians, it's essential to maintain our personal and professional boundaries while being open to multiple worldviews.

By establishing clear boundaries and being mindful of our biases, we can create a safe and supportive therapeutic environment for our patients. It's important to remember that we are there to support and guide our patients, not to judge or impose our own beliefs on them. Ultimately, our role as clinicians is to empower our patients to make their own choices based on their unique values and perspectives while also providing them with the necessary tools and resources to achieve their goals. By respecting our patients' boundaries and maintaining our own, we can work towards building a more inclusive, respectful, and effective therapeutic relationship.

As Novis-Deutch (2015) explained, both professions and religions have their own unique set of values, ideologies, and worldviews. Sometimes, they will clash; it is almost inevitable. Fortunately, research has demonstrated that individuals are able to commit to multiple worldviews, each with their own values, ideologies, and ideals, despite the fact that there may be some conflict between them (Novis-Deutch, 2015). As clinical professionals, it is our duty to establish multiple worldviews to increase our effectiveness and reach within marginalized and disparaged communities and populations while still maintaining our own sense of individuality and self.

Conclusion

Bias can be multi-directional, and when involving the religious traditions of the therapist and patient, it can be tricky to identify how bias manifests within the therapeutic process. This chapter has highlighted some of the ways in which bias can manifest based on the different possible therapeutic relationships involving religious and non-religious clinicians and patients. Additionally, the suggestions provided for bias resolution are in no way intended to be exhaustive. However, they are a good starting point to help the clinician diminish the negative impact that bias can have on the clinician-patient alliance. Further, suggestions on how to reduce the manifestation of bias are provided.

This chapter highlights the importance of traditional professional development methods, such as education and consultations, for addressing bias in clinical practice. However, it also emphasizes the significance of establishing and maintaining personal and professional boundaries as a critical component of professional development. The development of boundaries reflects professional growth and is just as essential as traditional methods for overcoming bias. It is important to note that boundaries should not be viewed as limiting, and clinicians should still strive to cultivate diverse perspectives while maintaining their own personal and professional boundaries.

References

Abernethy, A. D., & Lancia, J. J. (1998). Religion and the psychotherapeutic relationship: Transferential and countertransferential dimensions. *Journal of Psychotherapy Practice and Research*, 7(4), 281–289.

Byrne, J. S., Lack, C. W., & Taylor, K. J. (2021). Experiences of the non-religious in psychotherapy: Implications for clinical practice and therapist education. *Secular Studies*, 3(2), 187–205. DOI: 10.1163/25892525-bja10023

Duggal, C., & Sriram, S. (2022). Locating the sacred within the therapeutic landscape: Influence of therapists' religious and spiritual beliefs on psychotherapeutic practice. *Spirituality in Clinical Practice (Washington, D.C.)*, 9(3), 186–201. DOI: 10.1037/scp0000250

Grey, I., Tohme, P., Thomas, J., Mazrouie, M. A., & Abi-Habib, R. (2020). Preferred therapist characteristics of Muslim college women in the United Arab Emirates: Implications for psychotherapy. *Mental Health, Religion & Culture*, 23(9), 745–755. 10.1080/13674676.2020.1795823

Magaldi, D., & Trub, L. (2018). (What) do you believe? Therapist spiritual/religious/non-religious self-disclosure. *Psychotherapy Research*, 28(3), 484–498. DOI: 10.1080/10503307.2016.1233365

Novis-Deutch, N. (2015). Identity conflicts and value pluralism: What can we learn from religious psychoanalytic therapists? *Journal for the Theory of Social Behaviour*, 45(4), 484–505. DOI: 10.1111/jtsb.12079

Salem, S., & Hijazi, A. (2019). Does therapist–rater religious match predict higher therapist ratings? *Counseling and Values, 64*(1), 90–107. DOI: 10.1002/cvj.12096

Spero, M. H. (1985). *Psychotherapy of the Religious Patient.* Charles C Thomas.

Sue, D. W., Capodilupo, C. M., Nadal, K. L., Rivera, D. P., & Torino, G. C. (Eds.). (2019). *Microaggression Theory: Influence and Implications.* Wiley.

Trusty, W. T., Swift, J. K., Black, S. W., Dimmick, A. A., & Penix, E. A. (2022). Religious microaggressions in psychotherapy: A mixed methods examination of client perspectives. *Psychotherapy, 59*(3), 351–362. DOI: 10.1037/pst0000408

14

The Rewarding Journey of Working with Religious Patients

Introduction

Sex therapy with religious patients can present significant challenges. Yet, it can also be an enriching endeavor for clinicians, fostering personal and professional growth as they navigate the complexities of differing ideologies and worldviews (Singhal, 2016). While the confrontation with ideologies different from our own may be troubling, especially when they are counter to our professional opinions and perspectives, these experiences offer an invaluable opportunity to enhance our clinical skills. Engaging with religious individuals in the context of sex therapy requires therapists to develop a profound understanding of the specific religious beliefs and cultural backgrounds that shape their patients' perspectives on sex, sexuality, and relationships. It necessitates a delicate balance of respecting these deeply held beliefs while also addressing the patients' therapeutic needs. By cultivating this awareness and expertise, therapists can create a safe and inclusive space where patients feel understood, respected, and supported in exploring their sexual concerns within the framework of their faith. It's an intricate dance between the sacred and the therapeutic, but it holds the potential to foster transformative healing and growth for both patients and therapists alike.

DOI: 10.4324/9781003242017-19

For therapists, there exists a valuable opportunity for both professional and personal growth. The skills essential for effectively collaborating with religious patients are highly advantageous and have the potential to enhance our clinical expertise. As extensively discussed in this book, biases can easily emerge when engaging with patients from diverse faith traditions. Identifying these biases within ourselves and recognizing the multi-faceted ways in which bias can manifest within the therapeutic relationship serves as vital preparation for working with a wide spectrum of populations that clinicians might otherwise be inclined to reject or feel unprepared to assist. Within this context, an essential skill emerges the ability to cultivate productive working relationships with individuals holding differing viewpoints. In essence, it involves mastering the art of collaborating effectively with those whose opinions diverge from our own – a proficiency that proves beneficial not only within the therapy room but also in various professional collaborations.

Professional Growth

In the realm of sex therapy, a disconcerting trend has emerged wherein certain therapists decline to work with individuals holding differing worldviews. These perspectives encompass a spectrum of factors, ranging from political and religious to cultural and general attitudes toward sexuality and gender. It is crucial to challenge the notion that another person's opinions or perspectives are inherently harmful simply because they differ from our own. While they might provoke discomfort or even anger, it's important to recognize that divergence in viewpoints does not equate to harm.

Illustrating this point, I recall an encounter with a patient who sought assistance with issues related to his sexuality. Upon initial meetings, it became evident that he grappled with a profound conflict between his personal values and sexual orientation. Surprisingly, this struggle did not stem from religious or cultural beliefs but rather from political convictions. During one session, he asked if he could share a set of photographs with me, assuring that they contained neither nudity nor sexual content. As I perused the images, I found myself perplexed and uncertain about his intentions. The photo album featured pictures of him dressed in Nazi uniforms – a subject that inherently stirred discomfort within me, particularly as an Orthodox Jew practicing in Germany.

After a brief, uneasy silence, I inquired about the purpose behind sharing these unsettling images. He asked if I recognized their significance, to which I responded in the affirmative. Internally, I grappled with questions about whether he aimed to shock or offend me. The patient proceeded to clarify that he identifies as either homosexual or bisexual, while simultaneously holding strong Nazi ideologies, despite the fact that these ideologies oppose homosexuality. To reconcile these conflicting beliefs, he began the practice of dressing in Nazi attire and engaging in same-sex encounters, which has evolved into a significant aspect of his sexual identity. He states that this practice has now become a form of kink and something that he fetishizes.

Although I fully acknowledge the challenges associated with working with individuals who hold extreme racist, anti-Semitic, homophobic, or xenophobic worldviews, as clinicians, it is our ethical duty to offer care to those in need. While there may be differing opinions on this matter, it is a reasonable expectation for all healthcare professionals to extend their services to individuals regardless of their personal beliefs.

While professional organizations advocate for therapists to promote social justice, upholding ethical boundaries in these endeavors is crucial. Advocacy should never involve degrading, belittling, or attempting to re-educate those with whom therapists work. Additionally, ethical concerns could arise in the way that therapists advocate for certain populations as they often inadvertently disenfranchise others – especially religious populations. Wilson et al. (2017) shed light on the experiences of health inequity among marginalized communities, emphasizing the significance of understanding the differing worldviews between these communities and the healthcare providers who care for them.

Establishing Multiple Worldviews

As briefly mentioned in the preceding chapter, clinicians have the ability to develop multiple worldviews. In today's increasingly diverse society, individuals are often exposed to multiple worldviews through their professions, religions, and personal experiences (Novis-Deutch, 2015). This exposure can lead to the development of conflicting values and ideologies, resulting in identity conflicts and cognitive dissonance. However, there are strategies to navigate these challenges and establish multiple worldviews while reducing the potential for conflict.

First and foremost, it is crucial to acknowledge and respect the existence of different worldviews (Wilson et al., 2017). Actively seeking out information and understanding about diverse perspectives through reading, cultural events, and engaging in discussions with people from various backgrounds is essential. By embracing the diversity of worldviews, individuals can cultivate a more holistic and inclusive perspective that accommodates multiple ideologies.

Self-awareness of biases and assumptions is another vital aspect (Zhuang & Kong, 2023). Each person brings their own set of values and beliefs to any situation, and recognizing how these biases can influence perceptions of different worldviews is important. By actively challenging and examining these biases, individuals can develop a more open and accepting mindset toward multiple worldviews.

Effective communication skills are also crucial in navigating multiple worldviews. This involves expressing one's own views clearly and respectfully, while actively listening and empathizing with others. By creating a safe and supportive space for dialogue, individuals can foster greater understanding and appreciation of diverse worldviews.

It is essential to acknowledge that establishing multiple worldviews is an ongoing process that requires continuous effort and reflection. This entails being open to new experiences and perspectives and being willing to challenge one's own assumptions and biases over time. By committing to this process of self-reflection and growth, individuals can develop a more nuanced and comprehensive understanding of the world, minimizing the potential for identity conflict between multiple worldviews.

In conclusion, the study of religious therapists in Israel sheds light on the challenges of fully committing to multiple worldviews. However, by acknowledging and respecting different worldviews, being aware of one's own biases, developing effective communication skills, and engaging in ongoing self-reflection and growth, it is possible to navigate multiple worldviews and reduce the potential for identity conflict. This approach fosters a more inclusive and compassionate society that values diversity and promotes understanding across different ideologies and perspectives (Wilson et al., 2017).

Ethically Grounded Practices

As extensively illustrated in the preceding chapters of this book, the practice of working with religious patients consistently places clinicians at the crossroads of ethical dilemmas, transcending the boundaries of both the therapy room and their personal beliefs, or even the absence thereof. It is paramount for therapists to gain a profound understanding of their own biases and the myriad ways in which these biases can insidiously infiltrate the therapeutic alliance. This is a skill that is much needed far beyond the work with religious patients, but with all those who may seek help. Indeed, the ability to recognize and navigate one's biases stands as a cornerstone of effective and ethical therapeutic practice.

This fundamental skill extends its influence well beyond the realm of religious diversity. In a world where patients come from diverse cultural, ethnic, political, and ideological backgrounds, therapists must be adept at comprehending and addressing their own biases. Whether working with individuals from different faiths, political persuasions, gender identities, or social orientations, the capacity to approach each patient with empathy, respect, and an open mind is essential. It not only fosters trust and rapport but also enhances the therapist's ability to deliver culturally competent care.

Moreover, in an era marked by increasing polarization and societal divisions, therapists who can navigate these biases are better equipped to facilitate meaningful dialogue and healing. They play a vital role in bridging gaps, fostering understanding, and promoting inclusivity within their communities. Thus, the skill of bias recognition and management extends its influence far beyond the therapy room, serving as a beacon of hope and healing in an increasingly diverse and complex world.

This heightened self-awareness not only equips us to navigate the potential pitfalls when working with diverse patient populations but also empowers us to critically evaluate the recommendations we provide. It prompts us to discern whether our guidance genuinely serves our patients' best interests or is unwittingly swayed by our own subjective interests, ideologies, and convictions, ensuring that our therapeutic interventions remain objective and ethically sound.

Creativity in Therapy

Working with religious patients introduces distinctive challenges that demand a nuanced and creative approach. This context catalyzes the development of creativity in therapy as therapists navigate the intricate intersection of religious beliefs and sexual well-being. By crafting solutions that respect and honor the sacred tenets of their patients' faith while effectively addressing their sexual and relational concerns, therapists are compelled to think beyond conventional strategies, enriching both the therapeutic experience and the clinician's professional development.

Working with religious patients inherently invites therapists to embrace the richness of human diversity. It requires an open-mindedness that extends beyond the boundaries of traditional therapeutic modalities, challenging clinicians to consider a broader spectrum of solutions. This inclusivity expands their toolkit, drawing from a wider array of resources and approaches, ultimately fostering a more holistic and patient-centered practice. At the same time, it challenges clinicians to move beyond the realm of lazy solutions, which can hinder their therapeutic skills and professional development.

The delicate dance of integrating faith and sexuality forms the crucible in which creativity in therapy flourishes. Religious patients often grapple with a complex interplay of values, doctrines, and desires. This necessitates a customized approach that meticulously respects their belief system while nurturing their sexual well-being. Therapists, in this context, become adept at developing innovative interventions that bridge the apparent chasm between sacred teachings and intimate relationships. This capacity to harmonize seemingly disparate elements exemplifies the heights of creativity attainable in the therapeutic relationship. Within the pages of this book lie an array of illuminating case studies that serve as poignant testaments to the transformative power of working with religious patients. Each narrative provides a distinct perspective on how creativity was woven into the clinical process, assisting patients in discovering congruency between their religious convictions and their sexual health and overall well-being.

Sex therapy with religious patients provides a fertile ground for fostering creativity within therapy. This unique context prompts clinicians to push beyond traditional approaches, potentially reshaping the broader therapeutic landscape. Engaging with the intersection of religious beliefs and sexual well-being encourages therapists to explore innovative strategies, thereby enhancing their therapeutic repertoire and fostering advanced critical thinking skills. These gains, instrumental for professional development, empower clinicians to approach diverse cases with a more nuanced and effective therapeutic mindset.

Personal Growth

The challenges that commonly surface during the therapeutic journey, designed to provoke growth in those we serve, simultaneously challenge us. Our roles and interactions with patients constitute a two-fold influence, not only shaping our professional development but also molding our personal outlooks and attitudes. This phenomenon is not only observed when working with religious patients but also within the broader therapeutic context.

In Singhal's (2016) account, the researcher vividly illustrates personal growth as a therapist through the process of self-exploration and empathetic understanding. Singhal discusses the common struggle therapists face in empathizing with certain qualities or behaviors exhibited by their patients, especially when these aspects challenge their own comfort zones or ethical boundaries. In this particular case, the author provides an insightful example involving their work with a young patient named H, diagnosed with bulimia nervosa.

H's struggles with self-esteem, control issues, and self-destructive behaviors prompted the therapist to embark on a journey of introspection and self-examination. Initially, the therapist unintentionally reinforced H's progress, inadvertently pushing her to conceal her issues further. However, when H's father disclosed her secret struggles, the therapist grappled with feelings of failure and shame. It was at this point that the therapist's supervisor intervened, guiding them toward a more empathetic and non-judgmental approach. The supervisor emphasized the significance of empathizing with the patient's problems without categorizing her as either a "bad child" or a "model client."

Through this transformative experience, the therapist initiated a process of self-discovery and self-improvement. They recognized their own propensity to perceive achievements in an all-or-nothing manner, mirroring H's struggles with control. By confronting their feelings of inadequacy and acknowledging their own blind spots, the therapist gained a heightened awareness of their biases and limitations. Consequently, they were able to create a therapeutic environment where H felt validated and accepted, despite her setbacks.

Singhal's narrative powerfully illustrates how working with a challenging patient like H catalyzed personal growth for the therapist. This journey encompassed self-exploration, the development of empathy, and a shift in perspective, ultimately enriching the therapist's ability to provide effective therapy while simultaneously nurturing their personal growth and self-awareness. This experience exemplifies the concept of therapists and patients as "fellow travelers" on a journey of self-discovery and healing.

In a more recent article, Lin, Zhao, and Guo (2022) delved into the profound source of personal growth that dignity therapists encounter through the practice of Dignity Therapy (DT). Their study unveiled that engaging in DT offered therapists a unique opportunity for profound introspection regarding their personal philosophies concerning life and death. This self-examination, in turn, contributed to their psychological resilience, imbuing them with greater strength and empowerment.

Furthermore, the therapists participating in DT reported that it significantly enriched their lives in various dimensions. They gleaned invaluable insights from their patients' life stories, fostering a heightened appreciation for life's unpredictability and the importance of cherishing their own experiences. Learning from their patients' narratives inspired therapists to maintain an optimistic and positive outlook, even when confronted with adversity, encouraging them to seek meaning in their own lives, influenced by their patients' optimism.

The therapists also underscored the profound significance of family bonds and connections. Observing their patients' gratitude towards their families prompted therapists to cherish their own familial relationships and pay closer attention to these bonds in their daily lives. Additionally, therapists adopted a heightened awareness of health and well-being, recognizing the importance of embracing healthy regimens, guided by the wisdom and advice shared by their patients.

Additionally, Dignity Therapy exposed therapists to a profound understanding of their patients' suffering, thereby augmenting their capacity for empathy. While this heightened empathy occasionally led therapists to experience feelings of depression or distress when they couldn't effectively alleviate their patients' negative emotions, it ultimately contributed to their personal growth.

In both studies, Singhal (2016) and Lin, Zhao, and Guo (2022) provide critical accounts highlighting the phenomenon that engaging in therapy with challenging patients or using innovative therapeutic approaches can lead to profound personal growth for therapists. This growth encompasses self-reflection, empathy development, and a holistic perspective on life, underscoring the transformative potential of therapy for both therapists and patients, including aspects related to spirituality and religion.

Although research suggests that many therapists may avoid working with religious patients due to unresolved personal religious concerns (Magaldi, 2018), it's important to recognize that this challenge can also be an avenue for personal growth. Engaging with religious patients necessitates religious education, creative problem-solving, heightened cultural awareness, and often consultations with experts in the field. These experiences can serve as a pathway for clinicians to address and heal from their own unresolved religious concerns, contributing to their personal and professional development.

Healing from Previous Trauma

Sex therapists and psychologists frequently encounter cases involving patients who have experienced spiritual abuse or religious trauma. These issues often intersect with sexual and gender-related concerns, such as the role of religion in promoting conversion therapy (Plante, 2022). However, it's important to note that religious trauma, particularly associated with shame, can extend beyond matters of sex, sexuality, and gender. Some patients or clinicians may report experiencing shame rooted in past religious teachings, even if they never received explicitly negative messaging about sex.

Recent research by Donnie (2022) delves into the concept of religious trauma, especially within Christian contexts, and its connection to chronic shame. Although scholarly attention to this topic has been limited, religious trauma, characterized as profound psychological harm resulting from religious messages, beliefs, and experiences, is recognized as a significant contributor to mental health issues like depression and anxiety. The study emphasizes how religious trauma can accumulate gradually as individuals are exposed to messages that undermine their mental well-being, often tied to rigid emotional categorizations. It also points out that religious trauma can manifest as symptoms resembling post-traumatic stress disorder (PTSD), including intrusive memories and emotional disturbances, underscoring its importance for further research and intervention.

These findings are further supported by Ramler's (2023) article dealing with religious trauma. The author explores various ways in which religious communities and leaders can shape an individual's perceptions of sex, sexuality, and gender using biblical texts. Noting that many individuals may not even recognize the religious source of their trauma, with common symptoms including anxiety, depression, and a range of emotional difficulties. These symptoms may manifest as confusing thoughts, negative self-beliefs, decision-making challenges, a sense of isolation, and even PTSD-like symptoms like nightmares and flashbacks (Restoration Counseling, n.d.). Navigating such a complex array of emotions can be exceptionally challenging, especially for therapists dealing with their own mental health factors. Therefore, clinicians who have experienced religious trauma, whether related to sex, sexuality, or gender, must seek the necessary treatment to facilitate psychological, emotional, spiritual, and sometimes physical healing.

Being Open to Spiritual Development

Working with religious patients can provide psychologists with a unique avenue for personal growth through their own spiritual development. This journey can significantly enhance a therapist's professional competence and have a profound impact on their personal life. For instance, it has the potential to deepen the therapist's capacity for empathy (van Ments et al., 2018; Bauck, 2023), elevate the quality of ethical decision-making (Bauck, 2023), and cultivate a greater sense of optimism (Warren et al., 2015; Reynolds et al., 2019). Notably, increased optimism has also been associated with improved mental health (Laranjeira & Querido, 2022).

As clinicians engage in the process of understanding and respecting the religious belief systems of their diverse patients, they often become more open to personal spiritual development. This growth extends beyond the professional realm, enriching their personal lives as well. In this context, therapists begin to embody a more holistic perspective and approach to life, emphasizing the interconnectedness of personal and professional well-being. They may find themselves better equipped to relate to their patients on a spiritual level, fostering a deeper sense of understanding and trust in the therapeutic relationship.

Furthermore, this personal spiritual development can lead to a more comprehensive and nuanced understanding of the human experience. It allows therapists to appreciate the role of spirituality and religion in shaping individuals' lives and worldviews. This, in turn, enables them to provide more culturally sensitive and effective therapeutic interventions. By embracing their own spiritual growth, therapists can create a therapeutic environment that respects and honors the diverse spiritual and religious backgrounds of their patients, ultimately leading to more meaningful and transformative therapeutic experiences for both the clinician and the patient.

Conclusion

Working as a sex therapist with religious patients is undeniably challenging but offers substantial opportunities for personal and professional growth. Navigating diverse ideologies and worldviews, even when they diverge from our own beliefs, is crucial for honing clinical skills and expanding empathy and cultural competence (van Ments et al., 2018; Bauck, 2023). Understanding patients' religious beliefs and cultural backgrounds, striking a delicate balance between the sacred and therapeutic, can lead to transformative healing for both therapists and patients.

Professionally, therapists can acquire skills beyond the therapy room. Engaging with individuals of differing viewpoints fosters the art of effective collaboration (Warren et al., 2015; Reynolds et al., 2019). This skill proves invaluable not only within therapy but also in various professional collaborations, contributing to a more inclusive society (Wilson et al., 2017). Ethically grounded practice, recognizing and navigating biases, enhances cultural competence and bridges divides in an era marked by polarization.

Creativity in therapy emerges when working with religious patients. This context demands innovative approaches that respect religious beliefs while addressing sexual and relational concerns, broadening therapists' toolkits (Lin, Zhao, & Guo, 2022). Personal growth is an inherent part of the therapeutic journey. Through self-exploration, empathy development, and a shift in perspective, therapists undergo profound personal growth (Singhal, 2016; Lin, Zhao, & Guo, 2022). Healing from past trauma is also essential, emphasizing the importance of self-care for therapists who have experienced religious trauma themselves.

Ultimately, working with religious patients in sex therapy is a multifaceted journey demanding empathy, self-awareness, and cultural competence. It offers opportunities for growth on both professional and personal fronts, enriching the therapeutic experience for therapists and patients alike. By embracing these challenges and continually seeking personal and professional development, therapists can create a more inclusive and compassionate world that values diversity and promotes understanding across different ideologies and perspectives.

References

Bauck, P. (2023). Practicing neighbor love: Empathy, religion, and clinical ethics. *HEC Forum*, *25*(3), 237–252. DOI: 10.1007/s10730-021-09466-4

Downie, A. (2022). Christian shame and religious trauma. *Religions*, *13*(10), 925. DOI: 10.3390/rel13100925

Laranjeira, C., & Querido, A. (2022). Hope and optimism as an opportunity to improve the "positive mental health" demand. *Frontiers in Psychology*, *13*, 827320. DOI: 10.3389/fpsyg.2022.827320

Lin, J., Zhao, Y., & Guo, Q. (2022). Dignity therapists' experience of conducting dignity therapy with terminal cancer patients in mainland China: A descriptive qualitative study. *European Journal of Cancer Care*, *31*(6), e13670.

Magaldi, D. (2018). (What) do you believe?: Therapist spiritual/religious/non-religious self-disclosure. *Psychotherapy Research*, *28*(3), 484–498. DOI: 10.1080/10503307.2016.1233365

Novis-Deutsch, N. (2015). Identity conflicts and value pluralism: What can we learn from religious psychoanalytic therapists? *Journal for the Theory of Social Behaviour*, *45*(4), 484–505. DOI: 10.1111/jtsb.12079

Plante, T. G. (2022). The role of religion in sexual orientation change efforts and gender identity change efforts. In D. C. Haldeman

(Ed.), *The Case against Conversion "Therapy": Evidence, Ethics, and Alternatives* (pp. 109–124). American Psychological Association. DOI: 10.1037/0000266–006

Ramler, M. E. (2023). When God hurts: The rhetoric of religious trauma as epistemic pain. *Rhetoric Society Quarterly, 53*(2), 202–216. DOI: 10.1080/02773945.2022.2129755

Restoration Counseling. (n.d.). Religious trauma syndrome and faith transitions. Retrieved September 14, 2023, from www.restorationcounselingseattle.com/religious-trauma-transitions

Reynolds, J., May, M., & Xian, H. (2019). Not by bread alone: Mobility experiences, religion, and optimism about future mobility. *Socius: Sociological Research for a Dynamic World, 5,* 1–15. DOI: /1d0o.i.1o 1rg7/71/02.1317870/233718102938141980497

Singhal, M. (2016). Fellow travellers: A therapist's personal growth in the therapeutic process. *Asia Pacific Journal of Counselling and Psychotherapy, 7*(1–2), 133–138. DOI: 10.1080/21507686.2016.1213755

van Ments, L. I., Roelofsma, P.H. M.P., & Treur, J. (2018). Modeling the effect of religion on human empathy based on an adaptive temporal-causal network model. *Computational Social Networks, 5*(1), 1–23. DOI: 10.1186/s40649–017–0049-z

Warren, P., Van Eck, K., Townley, G., & Kloos, B. (2015). Relationships among religious coping, optimism, and outcomes for persons with psychiatric disabilities. *Psychology of Religion and Spirituality,, 7*(2), 91–99. DOI: 10.1037/a0038346

Wilson, D., Heaslip, V., & Jackson, D. (2017). Improving equity and cultural responsiveness with marginalised communities: Understanding competing worldviews. *Journal of Clinical Nursing, 27,* 3810–3819. DOI: 10.1111/jocn.14546

Zhuang, T., & Kong, X. (2023). Shaping personal worldviews when neo-liberalism meets Confucianism and patriotism: Insights from Chinese postgraduate students. *British Journal of Sociology of Education,* 1–16. DOI: 10.1080/01425692.2023.2195088

Appendix I: Glossary of Terms

Ablution (wudū') Ritual purification through washing before religious activities, often in Islam.

Ahl al-Kitab "People of the Book," referring to Jews and Christians in Islamic tradition.

Church Discipline Ecclesiastical measures taken within a religious community to correct or maintain behavior in accordance with its teachings.

Church Gossip Informal sharing of information, often about others' personal lives or behaviors, within a church community.

Cultural Empathy Understanding and appreciating cultural differences by putting oneself in another's cultural context.

Cultural Knowledge Awareness and understanding of cultural norms, values, and practices.

Cultural Responsiveness The ability to adapt and provide culturally sensitive care or therapy to individuals from diverse cultural backgrounds.

Cultural Sensitivity Recognizing and respecting cultural differences in attitudes, behaviors, and beliefs.

Ecological Systems Theory A psychological framework that examines how individuals interact with and are influenced by various systems or environments.

Exosystem In ecological systems theory, an outer layer of environments that indirectly impacts individuals.

Frum An observant or devout Jew who adheres to religious laws and practices.

Get A Jewish divorce document required to dissolve a marriage, particularly in Orthodox Judaism.

Hadd In Islamic law, a fixed punishment for specific offenses.

Halakhah Jewish law and legal principles derived from the Torah and Talmud.

Haram Actions or things forbidden in Islam.

Herem A Jewish ban or excommunication, often from the community.

Infallible The belief that a religious text is without any error or mistake.

Inspired The belief that a religious text was written under divine guidance or influence.

Interreligious Involving or relating to interactions between different religious traditions.

Intrareligious Involving or relating to interaction between the same religious traditions.

Ketubah A Jewish marriage contract outlining the groom's obligations to the bride.

Macrosystem In ecological systems theory, a broad cultural or societal context that influences individuals indirectly.

Madhabs Schools of thought or jurisprudential traditions in Islamic law.

Microsystem In ecological systems theory, the immediate environment or setting where individuals interact.

Mikveh A Jewish ritual bath used for various purification purposes.

Mitzvah A commandment or religious obligation in Judaism.

Mustakhbath In Islamic law, a person accused of committing adultery.

Niddah In Jewish law, a woman during menstruation period.

Nikah Islamic marriage contract or ceremony.

Pikuach Nefesh In Jewish law, the principle that saving a human life takes precedence over other religious obligations.

Polyamory A consensual romantic or sexual relationship involving multiple partners, with the knowledge and consent of all involved.

Polyandry A form of polygamy in which a woman has multiple husbands simultaneously.

Polygamy Marriage to multiple spouses simultaneously, including polygyny (one husband with multiple wives) and polyandry (one wife with multiple husbands).

Polygynandry   A mating system in which multiple males and multiple females form a multi-male, multi-female group.

Polygyny   A form of polygamy in which a man has multiple wives simultaneously.

Purgatory   A temporary state or place in some Christian beliefs for souls undergoing purification before entering heaven.

Rukn   In Islamic worship, an essential element or pillar of an act, such as the specific movements during prayer.

Salāt   Islamic ritual prayer performed five times a day.

Shahāda   The Islamic declaration of faith, bearing witness to the oneness of Allah and the prophethood of Muhammad.

Shariah (Shari'a)   Islamic law and moral code derived from the Quran and Hadith.

Taharat HaMishpacha   Jewish laws related to family purity and sexual conduct.

Tafsir   Islamic commentary and interpretation of the Quran.

Tarawih   Extra prayers performed by Sunni Muslims during the Islamic month of Ramadan.

Worldview   A comprehensive, foundational perspective that shapes an individual's beliefs, values, and perception of the world.

Zakāt   One of the Five Pillars of Islam, involving giving to charity and almsgiving.

Zina   Unlawful sexual intercourse in Islam, particularly outside of marriage.

Appendix II: Therapist Bias Reflection Questions

The following questions are provided to facilitate self-reflection, aiding in the identification and exploration of potential biases when working with religious patients. Additionally, these questions should help the clinicians consider other aspects of sex therapy with religious patients that they may not have considered. These questions do not aim to promote or endorse any specific viewpoint but rather serve as a tool for enhancing awareness of your own emotions, attitudes, and beliefs in this context. Think of these questions as being similar to those you may encounter in a Sexual Attitude Reassessment (SAR) workshop, allowing you to delve into your feelings, attitudes, and biases concerning religious patients struggling with sexual and gender issues helping you be more prepared when working in the therapeutic context.

1. How do you feel about the Bible being binary?
2. Does an adult have the autonomy to choose conversion therapy in order to align their sexuality with their spirituality?
3. Do you feel that sexuality is more important than religion? If so, why? And can you accept that a patient may hold a different perspective?
4. What comes to your mind when you think of fundamentalist Christianity?
5. Is it possible for a person to be sex positive while holding onto religiously informed boundaries?
6. Are you able to differentiate between religious trauma and a negative religious experience?
7. Can you recognize that a person can hold a different worldview than yourself without it being confrontational?
8. If a patient holds different values than yourself, can you recognize that they can be equally as important even if they are not a priority to you.

9. How do your personal beliefs and values, whether religious or secular, influence your approach to addressing the sexual concerns of religious patients?
10. Can you empathize with a patient's religious upbringing and the impact it may have on their sexual attitudes and behaviors, even if those beliefs differ from your own?
11. What are your initial reactions when a patient mentions religious practices or rituals related to their sexual concerns?
12. How do your own spiritual or religious beliefs (or lack thereof) influence your approach to therapy with religious individuals?
13. Have you ever felt discomfort discussing or exploring religious topics with your patients? What might be the underlying reasons for this discomfort?
14. Can you acknowledge the potential impact of religious guilt or shame on a patient's mental health and sexual well-being, even if you don't share their faith?
15. Are you aware of any assumptions or stereotypes you may hold about individuals from different religious backgrounds, and how might these impact your therapeutic relationship?
16. How do you navigate situations where a patient's religious beliefs conflict with widely accepted therapeutic approaches or interventions?
17. Can you distinguish between healthy religious expression and potentially harmful religious practices that may impact a patient's mental health or relationships?
18. What steps do you take to ensure that your own biases or preconceptions do not unduly influence the therapeutic process for religious patients?
19. How comfortable are you discussing sexual topics with patients from various religious backgrounds, and how might this impact the effectiveness of your therapy?
20. Are there specific religious practices or beliefs that you personally struggle to understand or accept? How do you work through these challenges in a clinical setting?
21. Can you empathize with a patient's experience of spiritual crisis, even if it differs significantly from your own beliefs or experiences?

22. How do you navigate situations where a patient's religious beliefs may be contributing to their distress or conflicts within their relationships?

23. Are you open to seeking additional training or education to enhance your cultural competence and understanding of various religious traditions, especially in the context of sex therapy?

24. How do you approach situations where a patient's religious beliefs intersect with issues related to gender identity or sexual orientation, and how do you ensure a respectful and supportive therapeutic environment for these individuals?

25. Can you describe a specific case or scenario where your own biases or lack of understanding about a patient's religious background led to challenges in the therapeutic process, and what steps did you take to address and overcome these challenges?

Appendix III: Helpful Resources

Training for Therapists

The School of Sex Therapy   OnDemand CE courses are available for working with all three Abrahamic faith traditions. Additionally, learners may opt to complete a certificate in sex therapy program with an emphasis on sexuality and religion.

Books

In the Footsteps of the Fathers: Psychosexual Therapy with the Orthodox Jewish Community – an Overview from the Therapist's Chair   by Judi Keshet-Orr & Sarah Collings

I Am for My Beloved: A Guide to Enhanced Intimacy for Married Couples   by David S. Ribner & Talli Y. Rosenbaum

Pure: Inside the Evangelical Movement that Shamed a Generation of Young Women and How I Broke Free   by Linda Kay Klein

Sex, God, and the Conservative Church: Erasing Shame from Sexual Intimacy   by Tina Schermer Sellers

Advancing Sexual Health for the Christian Client: Data and Dogma   by Beverly Dale & Rachel Keller

Organizations

Eshel   Eshel is a prominent organization that focuses on creating inclusive and supportive spaces for LGBTQ+ individuals, their families, and allies within Orthodox Jewish communities. They provide resources, support groups, educational programs, and host events that promote understanding and acceptance while respecting Jewish tradition. www.eshelonline.org/

JQ International JQ International serves LGBTQ+ Jews and their allies. They offer support, community events, educational resources, and cultural programs that celebrate the intersection of LGBTQ+ identities and Jewish faith. https://jqinternational.org/

Keshet While not exclusively for religious Jews, Keshet is a national organization dedicated to LGBTQ+ inclusion within Jewish communities. They offer resources, training, and educational programs that promote acceptance and understanding of LGBTQ+ individuals within various Jewish denominations. www.keshetonline.org/

Havruta: Jewish Queer Straight Alliance (JQSA) Havruta is an LGBTQ+ support and advocacy group for Jewish youth, particularly within Jewish high schools and universities. They aim to create safe and affirming spaces for LGBTQ+ Jewish youth to connect and discuss topics related to their identities and faith. https://havruta.org.il/

Believe Out Loud An online community and resource center that focuses on LGBTQ+ inclusion within Christianity. They offer articles, stories, and resources for LGBTQ+ Christians and their allies. www.believeoutloud.com/

Affirmation This organization is specifically for LGBTQ+ individuals within the Church of Jesus Christ of Latter-day Saints (LDS or Mormon) community. They provide support, advocacy, and resources for LGBTQ+ Mormons. https://affirmation.org/

Dignity USA An organization that advocates for LGBTQ+ inclusion within the Roman Catholic Church. They provide a welcoming community for LGBTQ+ Catholics and promote dialogue and change within the church. www.dignityusa.org/

The Reformation Project This organization advocates for LGBTQ+ inclusion within evangelical Christian churches. They provide resources, training, and a supportive community for individuals and churches seeking to become more inclusive. https://reformationproject.org/

Reconciling Ministries Network This organization works within the United Methodist Church to promote LGBTQ+

inclusion and equality. They provide resources for LGBTQ+ Methodists and allies. https://rmnetwork.org/

Muslim Alliance for Sexual and Gender Diversity (MASGD) MASGD is a national organization that seeks to support, empower, and connect LGBTQ+ Muslims. They provide educational resources, host events, and offer a platform for dialogue and advocacy. www.themasgd.org/

Salaam Salaam is an organization that focuses on supporting LGBTQ+ Muslims and their families. They provide a safe and inclusive space for LGBTQ+ Muslims to connect, share stories, and find support within their faith community. www.salaamcanada.info/

Podcasts

The Joy of Text Where Real Sex Meets Jewish Law – Hosted by Dr. Bat Sheva Marcus & Rabbi Dov Linzer

Intimate Judaism A Jewish Approach to Intimacy, Sexuality, and Relationships – Hosted by Talli Rosenbaum & Rabbi Scott Kahn

Sex for the Saints Hosted by Amanda Louder

The Natasha Helfer Podcast Hosted by Natasha Helfer

Sexvangelicals Hosted by Jeremiah Gibson & Julia Postema

Index

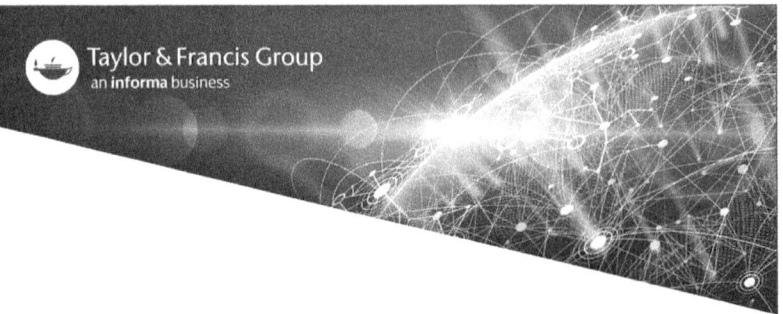

Taylor & Francis eBooks

www.taylorfrancis.com

A single destination for eBooks from Taylor & Francis
with increased functionality and an improved user
experience to meet the needs of our customers.

90,000+ eBooks of award-winning academic content in
Humanities, Social Science, Science, Technology, Engineering,
and Medical written by a global network of editors and authors.

TAYLOR & FRANCIS EBOOKS OFFERS:

A streamlined
experience for
our library
customers

A single point
of discovery
for all of our
eBook content

Improved
search and
discovery of
content at both
book and
chapter level

REQUEST A FREE TRIAL
support@taylorfrancis.com

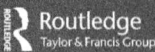

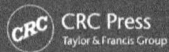